Preface

To you my dear reader, some words of advice from someone who's been there:

Are you frustrated that your body has not completely healed yet?
You WILL heal.

Are you struggling with the fact that you can never eat gluten again?
You WILL come to terms with it.

Do you dread going out to eat because of fear?
You WILL enjoy nights out again.

Do you feel like your life is consumed by this disease?
You WILL learn to live with it.

Do you feel awkward at social situations that are built around food?
You WILL realize that food is not what's important.

Are you jealous that others can eat whatever they want?
You WILL stop the defeatist attitude.

Do you just hate being a celiac?
You WILL learn to accept it.

Look…I get it. Our disease can consume us. Don't let it. We've got one life to live. Live it. And if you are struggling, just realize that many of us have been where you are now. Rest assured…YOU WILL GET THERE.

I promise you…celiac is not a death sentence. It's a life sentence.

This book will help you live that life.

FOREWORD: By Jennifer Esposito - My Friend & Fellow Celiac

(Dude note: I swear I didn't pay her to write this).

———

Being diagnosed with celiac disease after 20+ years of unexplained illness was actually a very happy day for me. I FINALLY had answers. What I didn't know is that the journey to healing had just begun. I may have had a diagnosis, but answers? Not so much. It seemed the medical community didn't really know what to say to someone like me who was having so many seemingly "unrelated" symptoms even after their prescription of choice, eating gluten-free. That is when I turned to the only people who spoke my language, the celiac community. I felt as though I had been dropped on Mars and finally found people that felt as lost as I was. We had the same pain, the same fears, the same struggle and mostly the same journey.

Enter Gluten Dude.

I was asked to speak at a gluten-free brand event about a year into my new celiac life. I was so happy to start speaking about all I learned and so wanted to help others struggling. I quickly realized that there was this slow rumbling that I could feel that was about to explode about "gluten-free" products, which meant lots of money for brands ready to offer these items.

With my very short time slotted on stage, 2 minutes I believe, the event suddenly became about gluten-free bread and NOT about the disease at all. I remember sitting with the gentleman in charge of THE brand and said, "I think you need to rethink your ingredients". I talked his ear off for about 45 minutes as to why. He just stared and nodded. He was frightened for sure.

You see at this point I knew that eating gluten-free was not enough and that we needed nutritious food to eat and be safe! But again I felt as though I was wandering alone though the forest with my ideas for health at this event that was geared towards making money.

Until — this nice, somewhat cautious, almost arrogant guy walked up to me and introduced himself as Gluten Dude. He told me that he had a blog and that he was moved by my story and wished he could have heard more of it. He went on to say that sadly many of these events aren't really about our disease and how to make a better healthier piece of bread, but rather more about making money.

Looking at me, almost judging my reaction, I remember thinking to myself, wow good for him!! He was the first person I had met at this point in my journey that was on the same page as I was. He took celiac disease as seriously as I did and knew the frustration it brought when others made it about something other than what it was, a disease.

He was also now looking at ME almost judgmentally, almost as if to say, "So what's your agenda?"

(Dude note: I really need to work on making a better first impression.)

He wasn't impressed by some "celebrity" talking about celiac, but more importantly what was my real goal now. Would I help or make things a lot worse for the community? He almost was standing at the gates, seeing if I was allowed in. He was actually protecting you folks, the celiac community, from more bullshit. I loved every minute of it. He then asked if he could interview me for his blog and I happily agreed. That day I went home and researched him and read his entire blog. I loved his attitude. I also saw that he pulled no punches with his interviews and I was ready.

To make this very long story a bit shorter, I braved his interview and on his next outing to NYC we set to meet up. We sat, also with his wonderful wife Deb, aka Mrs. Dude, and spoke for hours!!!! We spoke of our hard journeys, our fears, what we conquered and what we still had to overcome.

We spoke of food and the issue with the boxed chemicals we were offered and what we could do to help. **I liked these people; really liked them.**

Simply put, he was a human being, being human in wanting to help another who was struggling, because he had been there. That's it. No agenda, no big game plan, no scheme to make millions. Just wanted to help.

And he has.

The thousands who read his blog and also myself. He has helped me in more ways than I can write here and I am so happy that I was diagnosed with this crazy thing called celiac that day. If I hadn't been, I would have never met one of the greatest, greatest people, I'm so happy to call my dear friend in my life.

(Dude note: No I'm not crying…I'm just eating an onion sandwich, I swear.)

A Word from My Lawyer (Just kidding. I don't have a lawyer but please read anyway.)

I'm not a doctor. I've never played one on TV. Heck…I've never even stayed at a Howard Johnson's. My point? For ANY and ALL medical questions and issues, find yourself a good doctor. Yes, they can be few and far between but keep searching until you find one that will LISTEN to you. You don't want to get medical advice from a blogger, just like I wouldn't ask my doctor questions about running my blog.

To recap:
Got medical questions = doctor
Got questions about LIVING with celiac disease = I'm your guy

Introduction

Hi. My name is Gluten Dude. What's yours? (Isn't this how introductions work??)

I run a very popular blog over at GlutenDude.com. I've been at it since 2011 after my celiac diagnosis several years earlier.

Before we kick things into gear, I'm sure you have some questions. Like who I am *(a work in progress)*, why I wrote this book *(to help YOU)*, what you can get out of reading it *(peace, love and understanding)*, and most importantly, how it will help you kick celiac's butt. And kick it you will.

That's what the opening chapters are all about.

Enjoy.

Who the Heck is Gluten Dude?

Who am I? Darn good question. Been asking myself the same question since the day I was born.

As it relates to this book and my mission, I'm someone who's been gluten-free since 2007 due to a diagnosis of celiac disease, where the doc said my numbers were "off the charts". I'm someone who can steer you in the right direction when it comes to going gluten-free. And I'm someone who will always give you the naked truth about living with celiac disease. I didn't find freedom, a better life or any of that other crap when I got diagnosed. With all due respect to Hunter S. Thompson, I found fear and loathing of an unknown world. But if I can share my wisdom, tell my stories and make the transition easier on you, I've done my job.

As it relates to my celiac, I was actually one of the luckier ones. My symptoms were not as bad as many in the celiac community. I did not grow up feeling "sick" like so many others did. Although looking back, I now see a lot of health issues over the course of my life that I am convinced are celiac related. But for the most part, I was pretty normal (though my parents may seriously beg to differ!)

My main symptoms started about a year before my diagnosis and consisted mostly of constant stomach pains. Every night, I'd lie in bed complaining that my stomach hurt. And every night, Mrs. Dude would implore me to go to the doctor. And every night, I'd say "Oh…I'm fine." But after about a year of this, and losing 15 pounds on an already pretty slim frame, I decided to go to a recommended GI in Princeton, NJ.

Being the organized soul that I am, I kept a food journal for a week before my appointment. What did it consist of? A bagel here and there; a few bowls of pasta; a few beers. I thought I was being pretty healthy. The doctor took one look at my journal and my symptoms and asked me if I had ever heard of celiac disease. I had not. He said that I need to get tested ASAP.

The blood work came back first and he said they were the highest numbers he'd ever seen (I wish they said that about my SAT scores!!). He told me this as I was on the table about to get my endoscopy. So before I was put under, I pretty much knew. When I awoke, he said the villi in my intestine were pretty much gone and I indeed had celiac disease...quite badly.

And so my journey began. And what a journey it's been (and will continue to be). They say that life is not about what happens to you, but how you react to what happens to you. That, to me, is the key to adjusting to this insidious disease. You can let it beat you or you can fight it back.

This book is all about taking the fight to celiac. And winning the battle.

Why I Wrote This Book

Why am I writing a book at this time? What do I hope to get out of it? Who is it for? Lotsa questions…I get it. So let's get some answers; self-interview Dude style.

So you're writing a book. Why now?
Short answer? I want people to learn from the ups and downs and ins and outs of my celiac journey, which basically is what this book is.

Longer answer? I started my GlutenDude.com blog in October 2011. Since then I have written over 650 articles and the site has generated over 35,000 comments. I've written about a huge variety of topics, all regarding living with celiac disease. That's tons of material that needs to be seen by those in the celiac community who are looking for **honest guidance** (I don't sugarcoat things…at all).

The problem is that a lot of that material gets lost in the mix and may never be seen unless someone reads the blog from start to finish, and let's face it; no one has the time for that. And there are some seriously helpful / entertaining / important / educational / emotional articles that can benefit a lot of my fellow celiacs so they know what to expect and how to manage all aspects of their disease.

Although I have a pretty large social media and blog following, I know there are thousands upon thousands of fellow celiacs who have never heard of me or read my articles. So I am taking the best of the bunch, packaging up in easy to digest format and adding in a lot of new commentary as well. The bottom line is that I want to reach the biggest audience possible to ~~make as much money~~ help as many people as possible.

How would you say your blog, and hence this book, is different from other celiac related blogs and books?
Can we take a potty break?

No.

Fine. Like I said, I started my blog in October of 2011. Previous to my launch, I followed a lot of other gluten-free bloggers and I just felt there was a space that needed to be filled. There were, and still are, many talented bloggers in the celiac community. But the majority of them focus on the gluten-free diet aspect of the disease via product reviews, recipes, etc. I wanted to talk about the DISEASE and more specifically the realities of LIVING WITH THE DISEASE.

In addition, many of the blogs I read talked about how their lives drastically improved as soon as they gave up gluten. That certainly did not apply to my situation and I've heard from many celiacs over the years who have told me that it didn't apply to them as well.

So I wanted to be a voice that said *"Hey, you know what…celiac really sucks…here's all the crap we have to deal with…let's share our stories…find some sanity…get healthy…and make the journey together."*

So many celiacs in our community are lost. They get their diagnosis and the only instructions they receive from their doctor is: Don't eat gluten (thanks Doc). So we walk out of the doctor's office a bit terrified of our new life in front of us, but feeling a bit relieved that *"Hey…all we need to do is give up gluten and we'll be fine."*

But damn…here I am, 8 years after my diagnosis, and all I can say is that's just not the way it is. There is SO MUCH more to our disease than simply living gluten-free.

So you think you're filling a true need within the celiac community?
Absolutely. I would not write the book if I didn't. I realized that we need something that covers all of the emotional, social and physical aspects of living with celiac disease. We need something so that those newly diagnosed with celiac disease or those struggling with their disease have a go-to resource on how to best cope with their new life. We need something that is straight-up honest about our disease, with a lot of snark thrown in for good measure. We need something that tells celiacs *"hey…if*

15

...want to heal quickly...DO NOT make the same mistakes I made." We need...we need...we need...

THE NAKED TRUTH ABOUT LIVING WITH CELIAC DISEASE

Ok...I got it. So it's basically a handbook, or an instruction manual if you will, on living with celiac disease?

Exactly. This is essentially my journey through the ups and downs of this pain-in-the-ass disease. Look at it almost as a diary of my fun life with celiac disease. I'll provide specific guidance for those newly diagnosed and who are pretty much scared sh*tless...cause we've all been there. I'll talk about the pitfalls and how-to's of eating outside the comfort of your own home...and which spots to avoid even though they claim to be "gluten-free". I'll talk about how having the right attitude is an absolute necessity when dealing with celiac. I'll delve into how celiac can affect your relationships and how to navigate the sticky situations. And yeah...I'll even throw some celebrity juice in there, cause lord knows for the most part, they have not helped our cause.

How is your book formatted?

I struggled with how to organize the book. There is A LOT of content on my blog. I only wanted to bring the most pertinent information over. On top of that, my journey, especially when it comes to eating, has really changed over the years. As I put this book together, I realized in the beginning how much my blog was about my frustration with my disease, mostly because I was eating "gluten-free" and not eating "right". And yes...I've learned there is a huge difference.

So on top of focusing on how we should eat so we can heal, I thought it would be interesting to break each section down by topics (eating right, eating out, relationships, the right attitude, etc.) and for the most part listed by date as well. And where I want to add some current notes to an older article, I will mark them with "2017 Gluten Dude".

And one last item: My articles are really only a part of my blog. What makes my blog really shine are the comments on each post left by the community. As I mentioned above, over 35,000 comments so far. Even though the comments are so incredibly valuable and helpful (and pretty dang entertaining at times), I didn't want to add the comments to this book, so I strongly suggest you also visit my site and read through the comments. It's a true team effort in the Gluten Dude community.

Cool. Anything else we need to know?
Nope. Just sit back, get cozy, grab a gluten-free drink and we'll take this crazy ride together. Trust me...you don't want to go it alone.

You like me! You really, really like me!!

A little shout out in the title to Sally Field when winning the Oscar. If you don't know what that means, it just confirms the fact that I'm old. Anyway, I thought I'd throw in a few testimonials from my fellow celiacs. I don't do this to stroke my own ego (well…not really anyway). I do it so you can see that my blog and the GD community (and hence this book) has helped so many and can help you too. That's what I'm here for. (And by the way, that may be a total misuse of the word "hence". But I thought it made me sound mature, which is most likely a lost cause at this point.)

"Like John Lennon coaxing Prudence from her room, Gluten Dude asks other celiacs to come out and play. With acerbic wit, candor and a touch of rebellion, he's sharing his journey and he's enticing the celiac community to do the same."

"If you would have told me 18 months ago how blessed I would be by stumbling onto Gluten Dude's blog one frustrated day – I would have laughed and said "no way." Now, I sit here reading all these names I have grown attached to and think "HOW WOULD I DO IT WITHOUT THEM?" Their stories resonate with me and I don't feel like the odd woman out."

"I know I can't wallow and feel sorry for myself forever but I literally bawled my eyes out reading your blog because someone finally was being honest and understood and wrote the truth. So thank you so much!"

"Thank you – you beautiful soul – for providing the only place on the planet where I can sit in tears and say…damn this disease. It is the only place where with not an ounce of self-pity, we can just say FUCK THIS."

"Thank you, thank you, thank you. I can't say it enough. Your knowledge and honesty is like a life raft in an unknown and terrifying ocean."

"You have made me laugh and cry and everything in between and I'm only two weeks into your blog!!!"

"The blogs, comments and links from you and others in this community have given me much of my life back. Thank you!"

"I applaud you, Gluten Dude, for giving us Celiacs a place where we can chat, complain, celebrate and laugh at our all too real struggles."

"You just made me weep in the frozen food aisle of the grocery store while I wait for yet another prescription for our ever-sickly children! Thank you Dude!!!! You rock!"

"I had to let you know how much help your blog has been in getting my husband to understand better what it is like to have Celiac. For the first time in 14 years I found a place where I feel "normal". Thanks GD."

"I want to thank you for being so honest and supporting a gluten-free community that uses their knowledge and power for the good of the community. You are fighting the good fight sir and I appreciate you more than my words can really say."

"Thanks for the balanced approach, whether it is funny, sad, angry, silly or loving. We have all been through the emotional roller coaster. I look forward to hearing the real voices of the folks who comment here. You bring out the best in all of us! Thanks Dude!"

"I don't subscribe to your blog so that you can lie to me or convince me to try different products. I subscribe because your humanity shines through my computer screen and I think you are just like the rest of us......and on any given day that changes."

"You are like tonic to the gut, bubbling with humorous dialogue to cure the sad soul of any celiac needing attention. I am lifted from my moody mornings into hope for our future in a healthy community as I read your lines and the comments they generate."

"Thank you for always giving us information, sharing your experiences, and generally helping us all feel that we aren't crazy!!! I appreciate you, Dude!!! Keep up the good work."

"You make me smile, you make me cry, and you make me mad. But, most of all, you make me grateful that I don't have to figure this all out on my own."

"This blog just stopped me from going over the edge. Thank you!"

"This place feels to me the same way walking into the back door of my childhood home does…acceptance and understanding from my people!"

"Your take on things is amazingly refreshing. I learn more from you than from the dozens (hundreds?) of other gluten-free blogs on a regular basis. You done good, Dude!"

"I Googled "fuck celiac" and found my way to your blog. Thanks for blazing the trail. My life is better for your efforts."

"Gluten Dude, you really have impacted our two year ride with Celiac Disease. You reflect such a realistic view on this disease……while no one else understands, you and the people who gather here, make me feel just a little bit less crazy! THANK YOU!!!"

"Your latest post is why my son wants to be Gluten Dude when he grows up."

"I came across your Blog today and you had me in tears!!!! Tears of recognition that other people go through these frustrations, tears of laughter through understanding and tears of pain as I go through all of your contributors' rants and rages!!! THANK YOU!"

"Keep rockin' Gluten Dude. You are changing the world for us."

Rejected Book Titles

Before I decided on the final title of this book, I reached out to my awesome Facebook community and asked for some suggestions. I got 280 responses. Gotta love it. Here are some of the stand-outs.

- Celiac Disease: The Good, The Bad, The Poopy

- Celiac Blows

- Celiac Disease: Understanding the Misunderstood Condition

- Celiac Disease: Shootin' the Sh*t

- Celiacs Can Eat More Than Just Celeriac

- Celiac Disease: Managing Life In and Out of the Bathroom

- Celiac: The Nitty, Gritty, and Sh*tty

- Eat, Pray, Hurl – An Honest Account of Living with Coeliac

- Celiac Disease: Truth, Lies and Gluten

- Celiac Disease: The In's & Out's (LITERALLY)

- From Plate to Toilet: A Celiac's Handbook

- Celiac Disease: Do You Have the Guts?

- The Ryes that Bind

- Celiac – It's Not Just a Pain in the Ass

- Gluten Dude's Celiac Disease Survival Guide

- No…I Can't Just Eat a Salad!

- Pucker Up, Celiac Disease: Everything You Were Afraid To Ask and More?

- Gluten Wars: Return of the Villi

- Hold the Croutons!!

- Celiac. What the Bleep do I do Now?

- Celiac Disease: Fork Gluten

- Defloured

- Celiac Disease, No it isn't the Cool Trend

- Grab a Stool, Let's Talk Celiac

Yeah…they're a creative bunch!

Advice for the Newly Diagnosed (and Those Still Struggling)

Dude note: If you read nothing else in this book, please read this section, as it will help you avoid the rookie mistakes we all make and it will make the transition to your new life with celiac a hell of a lot easier.

The goal of this book is not only to educate and entertain, but to empower; to give those newly diagnosed the strength, confidence and knowledge they need to get busy living. To that end, I asked my celiac community the following question:

What advice would you give to the newly diagnosed? Not necessarily what foods to avoid because anybody can look that up. But what have YOU learned from living with celiac disease that you wish you knew when you were first diagnosed?

Here is some of the spot-on advice they offered:

- From day one, your illness will be trivialized. From the doctors who diagnose you, who can make it seem that going gluten-free is the easiest thing in the world, to anyone you speak to who tell you "there are so many gluten-free things on menus now, there's never been a better time to do it" (like it was a choice), to the waiters that roll their eyes at you. Rise above it.

- It is surprising and alarming how many food professionals have absolutely no idea what they are putting into their food.

- Some symptoms will lift immediately. For me, the migraines (which I didn't realize were related until after they stopped), the extreme bloating and pain ceased very quickly. Others will take a while. Be gentle. Know that your body will take a while to recover and that is OK.

- A lot of people go "Gluten Free" for weight and diet reasons. You very well could gain weight. I personally have been severely underweight for a long time. I gained 7.5 kilograms (16.5 pounds) when I stopped eating gluten. Roughly 15% of my body weight. Even though I was now eating a lot less, my body had not been absorbing what I had been eating. Weight gain was a very unexpected side effect!

- There will be a breakdown of some or many of your relationships. This illness can be debilitating and socially ostracizing. Either you will tire of the people who tell you how they eat gluten-free for "health reasons" and its SOOOO easy, or they will tire of you, because you are now a "burden" at social engagements.

- You will spend a lot of time apologizing for your illness. Over time you will stop doing this, but particularly in the beginning you will feel like a burden. Sometimes it's easier not to eat than it is to "cause a fuss." If anyone makes you feel like this – it's easier to remove them from your life than it was to remove gluten so feel free to do that.

- Research has indicated that there are significantly higher levels of depression and anxiety among those with Celiac Disease, in particular young adults. Celiac disease is 24 hours a day, with no end in sight. Most days it is OK, and you get used to it, but you cannot switch it off, you are constantly in a state of high alert, because anything that you put in your mouth can make you sick. More knowledge and awareness and comfort will lesson this, but it will never go away. Do not let it consume you.

- Check the ingredients of EVERYTHING. Gluten is a filler and hides in the most unexpected places. Some recent places that I have found it – Oral Contraceptive pill, Cold and Flu Tablets, and other medicines. Again – ignorance from medical professionals mean that you can and will still be prescribed tablets that contain gluten. Always always always double check.

- You WILL start to feel better. Your eyes will become clearer, the fog that you felt in your mind will lift, the migraines will end, the pain will end, any nutritional deficiencies you had will even out.

- There is something empowering about knowing that you don't have to take medication, and you can (to a large extent) control this illness.

- While you will lose some relationships, you will gain others. You will gain a new appreciation for people who have a basic respect and thoughtfulness for you, and the little things will become big things.

- There will be some long days, and hard weeks that turn into months, but you will discover a strength you didn't realize you had, and instead of feeling isolated, and isolating yourself, you will search deep into your own soul and the values of those around you, and surround yourself with people who make you feel exactly how you should – that celiac can suck, but it is not your fault, you are not a burden and you are not alone.

- Knowledge is POWER especially with this disease. I was diagnosed 6 years ago and I can say with 100% certainty that it does in fact get easier and better every single day.

- Attitude is everything in this journey and there's no other way to say it. Keep your chin up, don't apologize for having a disease that is out of your control and find new foods you enjoy that are also healthy for you.

- Stay away from the processed foods as much as possible. Fresh fruits and vegetables, meats, cheeses, wine, etc. are all gluten-free and fantastic! Keep it simple and learn to enjoy whole foods.

- You will link so many different problems to Celiac that arise. Issues that you thought were separate and just how your body works… good chance they're part of the effects of the disease. I thought

Celiac was mostly my dermatitis herpetiformus…turns out it's linked with fatigue, nerve and mood issues, insomnia, cramping, bloating, etc.

- It's a learning curve. Take it slowly and build on your knowledge base. You will make mistakes, and they will be painful. You learn from them though and move forward until it's second nature.

- It is so important to be your own advocate. If you think something is wrong, FIGHT for your doctors to hear you. I was almost not diagnosed because of my doctors. If your doctor isn't listening to you, it's time to find a new doctor.

- Life goes on, but gluten stays behind – You are going to feel angry, frustrated, and nervous after finding out you now can't eat some of your favorite foods, and while you may think "life as you knew it is over," you need to change your mindset and focus on what you CAN eat verses what you no longer can. It will make a huge difference.

- It takes TIME – Nothing comes easy or fast, and you'll realize that with this diagnosis. Patience is probably the hardest part because you just want to feel better NOW. Take it one step at a time, and know that things will start to become second-nature to you quicker than you thought!

- If you don't love cooking, learn to love it. Start experimenting with different ways to prepare foods that are very tasty to you. Also, don't take any food for granted. I made a lot of mistakes along the way eating foods that would normally be gluten-free but were not. Above all, be kind to yourself when you mess up and get sick. It happens to all of us.

- So many different symptoms with this disease, and sometimes, no matter how hard you try to do everything right, in the end, it is your acceptance that maybe you won't have perfect health with this disease which will help you the most.

- My contribution is to give yourself permission to grieve – the loss of your life as you now know it, the uphill battle with friends and family to come (*"No, Grandma, I can't use the same tub of butter"*), the radical changes coming your way (no more picking up Chinese takeout when you're too tired to cook). If you try to repress it at the beginning, you'll wind up standing in the middle of the grocery store, bawling your eyes out because you've just read a label and realized you can't have one of your favorite foods anymore. But it's just as important to move on from grieving – the radical changes coming your way DO include feeling better, knowing who your true friends are, and learning about lots of delicious food you might not ever have looked into (quinoa, anyone?).

- It may feel like your entire life revolves around food and eating safely. It may actually be true. Those with other illnesses/diseases have a heightened awareness about what makes them ill. Paying close attention to what you eat is no different. Think of it as saving your own life…your new mission.

- Advanced planning is part of your life now (as much as food is). Being spontaneous may be difficult but being healthy and having quality of life is so much better. Take a few minutes to pre-plan and everything else will fall into place.

- ALWAYS HAVE SAFE FOOD WITH YOU!!! Always. If there's an emergency you need to be able to eat safely.

- Learn how to say *"thanks, but no thanks"* to the well-meaning person who insisted they made you a special gluten-free dish for the potluck. If you know they understand cross-contamination, it's one thing, but for me the risk of getting glutened is so great.

- My advice is prepare for peer pressure. I don't mean stress about it. Just prepare yourself. Plan what you are going to do or say at the next company potluck when a coworker wants you to try his or her dish and even though they say its gluten-free, you watched three other people cross-contaminate the dish with the wrong spoon. Be ready for the next family dinner when Aunt Sally insinuates that a little gluten won't hurt anybody. From interactions to people close to you to complete strangers, have a plan. Write a list of things you can say. Keep your reasons short, polite, and to the point.

- LEARN TO COOK! You just have to. It's not that bad. And yes, you have the time.

- Know that a lot of the time you will feel like it's unfair. It is unfair that there are people who can be carefree and just walk into any restaurant and eat and you can't. But try to remember there are people who have it way worse than you. You can cure your body with just food!

- At the risk of sounding like I am trying to get on Gluten Dude's good side...the first thing I tell anyone newly diagnosed is GO TO THE GLUTEN DUDE website and meet your people!! I have told GD this but this website was a huge blessing and source of strength to me. The people here are amazing and made my life so much better. *(Dude note: I have a good side?)*

- There's a withdrawal. And it sucks. I'm pretty sure it feels just like going off sugar or caffeine. I felt restless, confused, I ate twice as much as usual for a week and never felt satisfied. Still, cold turkey is the way to go. "Easing" into the gluten-free lifestyle is only delaying the time you will feel better.

- You will find there are a lot of people spreading rumors, selling dubious products and tests, and just plain nonsensical "information" out there. You need to have a good dose of common sense, a basic understanding of anatomy, a basic understanding of cooking, and the ability to look for reliable scientific or medical information. Don't believe someone with a slick website calling themself a "gluten-free XYZ" or a "doctor of gluten" or some other made up credential.

- While it isn't a great thing to have this disease, having it will open your eyes as to what really is and isn't good for you, as well as teach you to be your own advocate and how to take care of you.

- You'll learn how to become a good advocate for yourself. It's hard – it's not something that comes naturally to many of us! But it'll get easier, and know that looking out for your health isn't being unreasonable, overly demanding, or "too needy."

- Socializing will be trickier for a while, but don't let your world shrink down out of fear. Sharing food is a central part of a LOT of our social moments, and it's going to take a while for you, your family and friends to figure out a new way of navigating these times.

- Grocery stores become grief stores. So much of what is sold is completely and forever off limits. Know this, and be ready for the weirdest bouts of grocery store tears. Once when the grocery store was out of my crackers, I wept, openly. This will happen, and its ok. After a while the tear portion of the program will taper off, and the angry section will open its doors. Losing so much food is bound to fire up the emotions. It's normal and you are totally allowed to express your feelings.

- Traveling by air and finding food either in the airport or on the plane is usually impossible. Carry your own, and more than you'd think is necessary. Supplement with chips, fresh fruits, and nuts, bought at the airport.

- Upon diagnosis, I cried, not because of the loss of all those foods I loved – I cried from sheer relief of finally knowing what my "enemy" was. The enemy had ravaged my body and nearly killed me. Focus on how good it's going to feel to feel good!

- Stand firm in your goal to become healthy. The enemy has been exposed and it is gluten! Now go fight for your health, and stop spending so much energy on the memory of those foods that robbed you of that health!

- And finally, never forget your sense of humor! Gluten Dude is an excellent example to us all. Keep pushing forward, never give up, and laugh at yourself and the tough things in life every chance you get.

And finally, here is MY biggest piece of advice. **Live Your Life.** Do not let celiac hold you back. It's a bump in the road, but it's a bump that is manageable. I promise.

Yes, you've got some serious adjustments to make.

Yes, your body will take some time to heal.

Yes, you will lose a little bit of freedom and spontaneity in your life.

But you know what? You're getting your health back and that's what matters.

There is an unbelievable amount of fear-mongering online. "You can't have this" and "you should stay away from that". Some of it is accurate. Some of it is complete BS. Stick with the facts.

Do not live your life afraid to do things simply because of GLUTEN. No matter what people say, it's NOT everywhere and you CAN lead a normal life (with a few adjustments).

Take precautions. Educate yourself. Use common sense. And if in doubt, do without.

And if you have any questions about something, just ping me. I'll set you straight.

Ok...let the fun begin! (That means turn the page.)

Chapter 1: Getting Defloured (aka How to Go Gluten-Free)

One word describes what it's like when you first learn you now have to live gluten-free. Over-friggin-whelming. But you know what? We've all been there. And you'll get where you need to be. When I was first diagnosed with this aggravating disease, I was angry, mad, pissed, upset. Pick a strong adjective and that was me. Six months earlier, I got a diagnosis of bladder cancer and now I had to deal with THIS?

All I could think about was the food that I could no longer have. My focus was not on my health, but on what I would miss out on. Not the best attitude I admit, but at the time, that's what I felt (and still do once in a while by the way).

I still remember going to Wegmans (our grocery store) for the first time after my diagnosis and just going up and down every aisle saying *"I can't have that. I can't have that. I can't have that."* It was so bizarre to me that all of the sudden there were so many foods that I could never eat again.

What seems almost impossible when you are first diagnosed becomes difficult; moves up to bearable; becomes manageable; and then eventually it just becomes the new normal. That's right…normal.

If you cannot stay 100% gluten-free, you will never feel "normal".

How do you get to that place? Let's dig in!!

Part 1: In the Head

It all starts upstairs.

So you just got the word you have to go gluten-free for life. I assume you've been diagnosed with celiac disease or a severe gluten intolerance. My condolences. As if your life wasn't challenging enough, you just got it kicked up a notch.

Right now, your head is spinning. What do I do? Where do I start?

Take a breath…relax…I promise you, while not easy, you can and will do this.

But before you go crazy emptying the gluten-free shelves at your grocery store (a typical newbie reaction, but also a big mistake), you need to mentally accept that you can never have gluten again. I will say it again…you can never have gluten again…ever.

It stings, doesn't it?

When I was first diagnosed, I remember telling Mrs. Dude that I can't make any promises I won't cheat. It just seemed so overwhelming. And permanent. And not knowing too much about the disease, I figured the occasional slice of pizza couldn't possibly harm me. Thankfully, I educated myself, I never caved and this allowed me to heal (eventually…after a long learning curve…which is why I wrote this book…no more ellipsis'…no seriously that's the last one).

But I know not everyone's will-power may be up to the challenge. Take my advice. Give yourself time. Not to eat gluten-free. That starts NOW. But mentally.

You're pissed…and rightfully so. It's ok to be angry. It's ok to mourn the loss of your old life. It's ok to long for the care-free days when food and spontaneity could be used in the same sentence. Be angry. Be sad.

But then move on. Look forward and not back. You have to or you'll lead a miserable, bitter life. You can't have gluten. Oh well. Face it…there are worse things in life. Much worse.

You have to rise to the mental challenge or you will never succeed in going gluten-free. A friend of mine recently stated over dinner that my disease must be great for my will-power. It is indeed. Once you get it through your head that you CAN do this, it really gives a jolt to your self-confidence that you can carry over to all aspects of your life.

So for the next few weeks, focus on brain-training. And I promise, eventually your mindset will shift and you will indeed transition from *"I can't have that???"* to *"I don't want that."*

And once you achieve that, you're half-way there.

Part 2: In the Heart

Guess what? You have to WANT to go gluten free.

I know. It sounds so obvious, doesn't it? I mean, of course you want to go gluten-free. You have celiac disease. You want to feel better. You want to stop taking 3 naps a day. You want to stop forgetting people's names. You want to stop spending way too much quality time with your best friend John.

But when you start to go gluten-free, you realize that *"damn…this is hard. Nobody told me it would be this tough to give up gluten. It will be so much easier if I sort of give up gluten."*

And that my friends is the beginning of the end for you. You will always cave to temptation. You will always be sick. And you'll always receive the scorn of Gluten Dude.

Going gluten-free is all about embracing your new lifestyle.

You've been dealt a pretty shitty hand. Accept it. Embrace it. Take all the negative emotions associated with the many crappy things that come with celiac disease and turn them into positives.

I can't have pasta? I want to try corn, rice or black bean pasta (I really recommend that last one!).

I can't have bread? I want to avoid the empty calories it provides anyway.

I can't drink beer? I want to start dabbling in red wine.

I can't have pizza? I want to try to make my own healthier alternative.

I can't have Chinese food? I want to start eating sushi.

And guess what? Your new life will be better. Face it. You've most likely been living the same life, making the same decisions and eating the same foods for your entire life. If you think about it, it's kinda boring. You've got an opportunity to completely change how you live. I think that's pretty cool.

Want it. Accept it. Embrace it. Live it.

Part 3: In the House

Be the master of your domain

It's pretty easy to keep gluten out of most of the rooms in your house.

The bedroom? Unless you're into some unusual practices (none of my business), I'd say it's pretty safe.

Bathroom? Should be good.

Family room? Iffy if you've got kids, but not too bad.

But the kitchen? Unless your entire house is gluten-free, this is where the majority of the nasty gluten critters will be lurking. If you're going to get cross-contaminated, odds are it's gonna happen here. Hate to break it to you, but you need to keep your kitchen clean, uncluttered and safe. The less clutter, the less chance for cross-contamination.

Keep your kitchen as gluten-free as possible.

1. Buy separate kitchenware for your use only. Everything we bought was red to make it easier to differentiate. Things you'll need include your own toaster, cutting board, colander and pots and pans. Yep…it's expensive to have celiac.

2. Have one counter in your kitchen completely gluten-free at all times. It should be off limits to anybody but you. Kinda nice actually. Feel a bit like royalty.

3. Keep your food separate from food with gluten. In the fridge and freezer, you should have your own shelf. In the cabinets, if you have a big enough kitchen, try to get one cabinet that is just your food. It makes it so much easier when things are separated.

4. Get a different colored sponge for your gluten-free dishes. Again, do red to keep it consistent.

5. Put "gluten-free" stickers in any location where there is no gluten allowed. This especially helps when you have company.

6. Make sure your family is 100% on board and knows the rules of the kitchen. And trust me, getting your teen to stop cutting her bagels on my friggin' counter is easier than it sounds.

7. Be patient and always, always, always err on the side of caution.

May the gluten-free gods be with you.

Part 4: In the Restaurant

Out to eat? Play it safe. Really, really safe.

When you've got celiac disease, going out to eat sucks. I wish I could sugarcoat it for you a little bit, but there are just no two ways around it.

Why does a normal person go out to eat? To try new foods. To eat in a different atmosphere. To get waited on. To steal from your kid's plates when they're not looking.

But almost everything that is fun and spontaneous about eating out can be overshadowed by the anxiety of whether you can get through your ordeal unscathed.

Will your server be understanding/patient/human?

Will the kitchen know what you're talking about when you try to explain what gluten is?

Will they take it as seriously as you need them to take it?

Do they *really* understand about cross-contamination?

And lastly, will you have your next six months ruined because you just wanted to get out of the house for an evening?

So what's a poor celiac do to??

The following are the steps I took on a recent night out to a restaurant I had never been to before. Do the same and increase your odds of a healthy, happy evening.

Step 1: A few hours before we left, I **called the restaurant** and asked to speak with the manager (who sounded about 12...first bit of trepidation). I explained my situation and I was told they actually had a gluten-free menu. That's a good sign, but not a guarantee they have their sh*t together.

Step 2: As we entered the restaurant, I again asked to **speak with the manager** just to say *"Hey…I'm the guy who called. Please be my friend tonight."* We went over the menu a bit and I took my seat.

Step 3: While everyone else looks at the menu to see what they want, I **study the menu** to see what I cannot have (which is usually about 95% of the menu). It's a process of elimination that can take some time. If it's a large menu, sometimes I don't even bother and I just wait until the server comes along.

Step 4: The server comes over to the table and I stand up and **quietly explain my situation** to her. Note that I said quietly. I hate the attention that my situation brings and I also don't want to put the waitress on the spot in front of the whole table. We go over the do's and don'ts and the can's and can'ts of making my meal safe.

Step 5: It's time to order. The moment of truth. I usually have at least three items that I will ask questions about and will **always go with the safest choice**, even if it's not my first choice. I get the Ahi Tuna with no sauce, veggies and brown rice. A bit nervous about the rice, but she assures me it's ok.

Then she asks if I want the soup with my dinner. Of course I say no, but she says it's vegetarian chili and it's totally safe for me to eat. At this point, I had a weak moment. I said ok. Stupid, stupid, stupid. Too many ingredients. Too many things that can go wrong. The risk far outweighed the reward. Mrs. Dude wasn't a happy camper. And rightfully so. I did not practice what I preach.

So is the extra work/worry worth it? Are you better off just staying home? I can't answer that. From a health perspective, you put yourself at risk anytime you eat food that someone else prepares. But at the same time, we have to live our life, right?

Just don't order the chili.

Part 5: Now What?

Ok…now what happens?

Am I mentally prepared to go gluten-free? Check.

Am I emotionally committed to a gluten-free life? Check.

Is my house a gluten-free sanctuary? Check.

Will I be my own best advocate when going out to eat? Check.

Well…you're off to a great start. You are indeed way ahead of the game. And I wish I could say it's all downhill from here, but the truth is, my friend, your journey has just begun.

Every day is a gluten-free challenge…

It's monotonous talking about gluten all the time. It's annoying checking Google three times a day to see if something has gluten in it. It's frustrating watching everybody else eat whatever they want while your choices seem so limited. It's painful not being able to eat Mrs. Dude's Rum Cake (you have no idea how sinfully delicious it is.)

Let's face it. It can pretty much suck.

…but you will prevail.

Why? Because you're smart. You're strong. You're disciplined.

And if you want to live a long, healthy life, you simply have no choice.

I was at a friend's house last night and our lovely host was telling me about another friend of hers who has celiac, but "she isn't as careful as you are." Part of me felt bad for her, as I know what is happening to her insides every time she cheats, whether she feels sick or not. But another part of me felt angry. If you're gonna play that game, then you know what, don't tell people you have celiac disease. If you're gonna cheat once in a while, keep your disease to yourself, as it makes people like me who treat it as a life or death situation look like we're hypochondriacs.

You will not be that person. You cannot be that person. You understand me?

You've got a long, wonderful gluten-free life ahead of you.

Enjoy it. Savor it. And if you're ever in a moment where you feel you might break, ping me, and I'll talk you off the ledge.

Chapter 2: Living With Celiac Disease – The Nitty, the Gritty and the Sh*tty

Ah…this wonderful disease they call celiac. *Just go gluten-free* they all said *and you'll feel better right away*. Yeah right. One thing I did not know about celiac is how it encompasses your entire life. I don't mean that it's always difficult or I always hate it or I struggle with it daily. I just mean that you can never forget you have celiac disease. It is a constant (unwanted) companion.

What does it mean to "live with celiac"? It means dealing with symptoms that at first seem to have nothing to with celiac disease. It means dealing with false narratives and fear-mongering. It means dealing with food companies that may not have your best interest in mind. It means dealing with…LIFE.

I've written so many posts about living with our disease. Some personal, some observational and all brutally honest. Hopefully, they will help YOU live a better life.

Celiac Disease Symptoms (from Those Living with the Disease)

2017 Gluten Dude: The following infographic was made back in 2012 and has been shared thousands of times, has been added to several doctors's offices, was in a newspaper, has been translated into various languages, and (pathetically) it's even been stolen by people who claim it as their own. I've had people email me that seeing this saved their lives as they were dying inside and never would have suspected celiac. While it doesn't say much for our medical community, it still warms my heart that it's helping people. Feel free to pass it along (hi-res and in color), using this link: https://glutendude.com/celiac-disease-symptoms.jpg

I think most of us will agree that the medical community is just a tad behind when it comes to fully understanding celiac disease symptoms. We have heard plenty of doctor horror stories to attest to this. And the internet can make things just as confusing.

On one side of the spectrum we have the websites who list the celiac disease symptoms as simple digestive issues: stomach ache, bloating, etc. Yes, that plays a large part but we all know it goes WAY beyond that.

And on the other side we have the sites that list hundreds of possible celiac disease symptoms, which may indeed be the case but it doesn't say which ones are the most common and which ones could be a stretch.

And I believe that most of these websites get the list of symptoms from the medical community.

I wanted to do things a bit differently. I thought it would be extremely helpful to get a complete list of celiac disease symptoms directly from the best source possible: those suffering with this disease.

So I asked the community *"what are your celiac symptoms?"* and their responses (as usual) were fantabulous.

To make the list of celiac symptoms as accurate and easy to read as humanly possible, without listing every single possible symptom, I only listed those that were mentioned by more than one person. And the symptoms that were mentioned the most often were given extra prominence. And on top of that, I broke the symptoms down by category.

And after all this effort, wouldn't it be nice to come up with something a bit different? A bit more visual?

So I got my creative juices flowing. The result is the following infographic:

WHAT ARE THE SYMPTOMS
OF CELIAC DISEASE?

HAVE THESE SYMPTOMS? DON'T WAIT. GET TESTED.

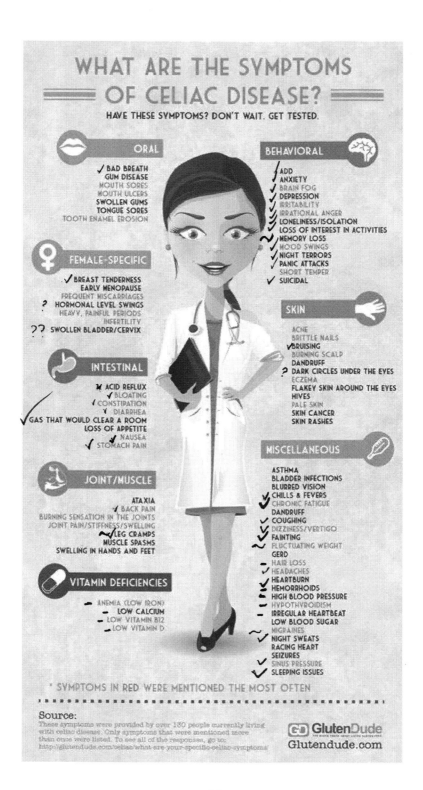

ORAL
- ✓ BAD BREATH
- GUM DISEASE
- MOUTH SORES
- MOUTH ULCERS
- SWOLLEN GUMS
- TONGUE SORES
- TOOTH ENAMEL EROSION

FEMALE-SPECIFIC
- ✓ BREAST TENDERNESS
- EARLY MENOPAUSE
- FREQUENT MISCARRIAGES
- ? HORMONAL LEVEL SWINGS
- HEAVY, PAINFUL PERIODS
- INFERTILITY
- ?? SWOLLEN BLADDER/CERVIX

INTESTINAL
- ✗ ACID REFLUX
- ✓ BLOATING
- ✓ CONSTIPATION
- ✓ DIARRHEA
- ✓ GAS THAT WOULD CLEAR A ROOM
- LOSS OF APPETITE
- ✓ NAUSEA
- ✓ STOMACH PAIN

JOINT/MUSCLE
- ATAXIA
- ✓ BACK PAIN
- BURNING SENSATION IN THE JOINTS
- JOINT PAIN/STIFFNESS/SWELLING
- ✓ LEG CRAMPS
- MUSCLE SPASMS
- SWELLING IN HANDS AND FEET

VITAMIN DEFICIENCIES
- – ANEMIA (LOW IRON)
- – LOW CALCIUM
- – LOW VITAMIN B12
- – LOW VITAMIN D

BEHAVIORAL
- ✓ ADD
- ✓ ANXIETY
- ✓ BRAIN FOG
- ✓ DEPRESSION
- ✓ IRRITABILITY
- ✓ IRRATIONAL ANGER
- ✓ LONELINESS/ISOLATION
- LOSS OF INTEREST IN ACTIVITIES
- ✓ MEMORY LOSS
- MOOD SWINGS
- ✓ NIGHT TERRORS
- ✓ PANIC ATTACKS
- SHORT TEMPER
- ✓ SUICIDAL

SKIN
- ACNE
- BRITTLE NAILS
- ✓ BRUISING
- BURNING SCALP
- DANDRUFF
- ? DARK CIRCLES UNDER THE EYES
- ECZEMA
- FLAKEY SKIN AROUND THE EYES
- HIVES
- PALE SKIN
- SKIN CANCER
- SKIN RASHES

MISCELLANEOUS
- ASTHMA
- BLADDER INFECTIONS
- BLURRED VISION
- ✓ CHILLS & FEVERS
- CHRONIC FATIGUE
- DANDRUFF
- ✓ COUGHING
- ✓ DIZZINESS/VERTIGO
- ✓ FAINTING
- ✓ FLUCTUATING WEIGHT
- GERD
- HAIR LOSS
- ✓ HEADACHES
- ✓ HEARTBURN
- ✓ HEMORRHOIDS
- ✓ HIGH BLOOD PRESSURE
- HYPOTHYROIDISM
- IRREGULAR HEARTBEAT
- LOW BLOOD SUGAR
- MIGRAINES
- ✓ NIGHT SWEATS
- RACING HEART
- SEIZURES
- SINUS PRESSURE
- ✓ SLEEPING ISSUES

* SYMPTOMS IN RED WERE MENTIONED THE MOST OFTEN

Source:
These symptoms were provided by over 180 people currently living
with celiac disease. Only symptoms that were mentioned more
than once were listed. To see all of the responses, go to:
http://glutendude.com/celiac/what-are-your-specific-celiac-symptoms

GlutenDude
Glutendude.com

What it's Truly Like to Have Celiac Disease

I once received an email from somebody asking how he should best respond to his girlfriend, who has celiac disease, when she does not feel well. I opened the question to the forum and as usual, the community rocked with their responses. But there was one comment from Miss Dee Meanor (love the name!) which just totally captured the essence of celiac disease in a way I could not communicate as I continue to struggle with this affliction.

I was so blown away by her response that I asked her if I could make her comment its own blog post to give people a vivid portrayal of our disease. She complied. Here it is.

"

So many times we look okay on the outside and no one can see the bone-weary tiredness, the aching joints, the fuzzy brain, and/or the war going on inside our bodies. We go to work when we don't feel well because we have to. Our sick leave is reserved for times when we simply can't function at all or for the multitude of doctor visits that are sure to arise from other complications caused by the disease.

Our "tired" when we're glutened is not the same "tired" that you feel. There should really be a new word invented for the "gluten tired" that makes it a Herculean task just to walk through the house.

Don't feel offended if she seems fine with people outside the home and then sick when she returns home.

We often smile and chat with people because we feel we have to. Sometimes our jobs depend on it. Sometimes we have social occasions that we must attend and don't want to be the guest that dampens the entire occasion. (i.e. weddings, business dinners, family holiday celebrations).

When we come home, we are spent physically and emotionally. It takes a toll on everyone, but especially loved ones who get the short end of the physical and emotional stick. In other words, know that we become good at smiling through the pain for others because we have to, but appreciate NOT having to do that with the ones we love. She thanks you for allowing her to feel safe enough to drop the act when she is with you. Sadly, many of us have loved ones that take offense and feel they are being treated worse than strangers.

Don't take offense if she doesn't want to be touched at all. Know that sometimes a gentle hug or caress can hurt. My husband loves to put his arm around my waist, but if I've been "glutened" I will flinch and draw away as a reflex. What he can't see is that I feel like my abdomen is an overinflated balloon. I have even looked in the mirror sometimes thinking I must look six months pregnant and am surprised to see that I look no different. The best thing is for the two of you to open the communication lines.

We actually joke about what my husband calls the "Don't touch the tummy!" moments.

Know that advance plans are scary for us because we never know from day-to-day how we're are going to feel. That event scheduled two months from now can't be fully appreciated until the day before. I've actually been a paranoid basket case just before an event and have eaten next to nothing. We simply can't get as excited at events on the calendar as others. It isn't because we aren't excited to do things with you. We are afraid that we're going to feel horrible on that date and don't want to disappoint you.

Sometimes things that are exciting for most people like cruises, resorts, and multiple destinations are scary for us. Buzzwords like "all-inclusive" are particularly horrifying because we're locked in to where and what we eat. Part of the fun for any trip is sharing meals. Unfortunately, for us that becomes the biggest stress and fear. Throw in a trip where we don't speak their language and the fear is magnified.

Be willing to be flexible. One crumb can make that dream vacation or even dinner and a movie become months of torture. One vacation in San Diego I ate dinner at one location I knew to be safe and then we went to another for my husband to eat at his favorite Mexican eatery. We still had a great time.

Be her champion. My husband is now a pro at questioning restaurant staff and talking to managers when I feel like I just can't talk about gluten or cross-contamination another moment. He is my second set of eyes for little things like spoons being double-dipped from gluten items into the gluten-free ones. He educates others. He doesn't ask what he can do to help because he knows I hate being an invalid. Instead he says, "Let me do that for you." (Those six little words say more than all the Hallmark cards ever written.)

"

In a Word, What is Celiac Disease?

Boo! Celiac Disease is **Frustrating**
Just when you start to feel better, something seems to inevitably happen to bring you back down. And most of the time, you have no idea what it was.

Yay! Celiac Disease is **Healthy**
Because you can't eat gluten, it removes so many unhealthy options from your diet (as long as you don't replace them with equally unhealthy choices as most newly diagnosed celiacs do).

Boo! Celiac Disease is **Expensive**
Your own cookware, your own utensils, gluten-free food that is double the price of normal food for no apparent reason, and the list goes on.

Yay! Celiac Disease is **Empowering**
If you can maintain a 100% gluten-free diet, which is soooo not easy, it makes you feel like you can accomplish anything.

Boo! Celiac Disease is **Time-consuming**
Say good bye to spontaneity. On the road and getting hungry? Good luck with that one.

Yay! Celiac Disease is **Ego-boosting**
Your own kitchen counter; your own shelf in the fridge; your own cabinet. How cool is that?

Boo! Celiac Disease is **Painful**
Sometimes, the disease just hurts.

Yay! Celiac Disease is **Cleansing**
Lots of time spent in the bathroom…ummm…flushing out your system.

Boo! Celiac Disease is **Limiting**
Out of a four page restaurant menu, you can have only a handful of items…if that.

Yay! Celiac Disease is **Social**
The celiac community is filled with wonderful people who really seem to want to help others in their situation.

Boo! Celiac Disease is **Life-threatening**
If you are misdiagnosed or do not follow a strict gluten-free diet, your body will seriously pay the price.

Yay! Celiac Disease is **Manageable**
There are many diseases more serious than celiac disease. Trust me folks…it could be a lot worse!

Celiac Disease: A Day in the Life

> 2017 Gluten Dude: This article was written before I completely overhauled my diet. I cringe looking back at how I used to eat. No wonder I never felt well. Gorilla Munch? Udi's bagel? Have not touched them in years. You live and you learn. And I'm so glad I learned (and still living by the way.)

Ever wonder what it's like to have celiac disease? Of course you do. Let me take you through 24 hours of my life and see what a pain in the ass, I mean what a joy it is to have celiac.

7:00am: Wake up. Crave coffee. Make coffee. Drink coffee. So far, so good.

7:30am: My first hunger pang. Luckily, breakfast is probably the easiest meal to figure out. Plenty of good gluten-free cereals on the market. Pour a bowl of Gorilla Munch with almond milk. Half-way thru meal, stomach hurts already. Dump the rest out. *On a side note, I once offered my daughter's friend some Gorilla Munch and she was absolutely horrified. Note to company: perhaps not the best choice for the name of a food.*

7:40am: Bathroom trip. Will spare you the details.

12:00pm: Make lunch. 3 eggs and an Udi's bagel. Forget to put the toaster on the bagel setting and burn the crap out of my bagel. Rats. Eat it anyway.

12:40pm: All packed and ready to go for an overnight in Philly (30 minutes away). We have a charity event to attend.

12:41pm: Realize I haven't packed any food for my journey. Open my gluten-free drawer and throw a potpourri of items in a bag: Twigs & Sticks, 3 bananas, 2 Kind bars, almonds and pistachios. Way to plan ahead Dude.

3:00pm: Arrive in Philly and immediately think food. Simply cannot risk eating out and ruining my night (and next six months) by getting glutened. Play it safe and get some sushi (the Dude's favorite).

5:00pm: Go up to the top floor of hotel for some free appies and beverages. Everything looks awesome. And dangerous. I ask the server if the tuna is ok. She checks with the chef. Says it's fine. Gives me ingredients. Includes soy sauce. Sigh. Watch everyone else eat.

6:30pm: Arrive at charity event. Cocktail hour first. Wow…everything looks great. I eat a carrot. Head to the bar.

8:00pm: First dinner course is served. We planned ahead to let the hotel know my dilemma but the server seems really annoyed when I remind him. Brings salad out. Looks dangerous. Remind him AGAIN I cannot eat gluten. Takes salad back. Brings back a plate of lettuce. Head back to bar.

9:00pm: Main course. Steak and shrimp over a sweet potato puree. As long as I don't have the sauce on top, server assures me it's totally safe. Must eat so I have no choice. Really good, but hard to enjoy as I just can't be sure it's ok.

10:00pm: Dessert served. Not even close.

1:00am: Back at the hotel lobby. Everybody drinking. Everybody starving. Somebody goes out and brings back 20 slices of all kinds of pizza. Everybody enjoys. Well, not everybody.

2:00am: Call it a night. Already mourning the next morning's breakfast that I won't be able to eat.

9:00am: Breakfast. Everyone complaining about all the crap they ate the night before. I eat my fresh fruit and smile.

Hmmm…maybe having celiac isn't so bad after all.

9 Signs You May Have Celiac Disease

Drum roll please…

1. You spend half your day in the bathroom and the other half making sure you are near a bathroom.

2. People ask you when the baby is due…and you're a guy.

3. After eating Thanksgiving stuffing, you don't make it out of bed until Sunday.

4. You drink half as many beers as your friends, but feel twice as sick in the morning.

5. You constantly start sentences but because of brain fog…

6. You have what looks like poison ivy…and you live in Manhattan.

7. You've been misdiagnosed as having IBS, Crohn's, anemia and an ulcer…all by the same doctor.

8. You eat more than ever, but people are always asking you if you've lost weight.

9. You nap more than a two year old.

What's it Like to be Glutened?

In a word? UGLY.

A little background first. I got diagnosed in 2007 with severe celiac disease. On day 1 of my diagnosis, I went gluten-free and never looked back. Actually, that's not true. I looked back a lot; but never gave in to temptation.

Fast forward 3.5 years. I am out with Mrs. Gluten Dude at a sushi restaurant to remain nameless. (But if I were to give it a name, I would call it A-1 Sushi in Langhorne PA.)

Now as most of you celiacs know, going to a new restaurant is an adventure in fear and anxiety. Really takes about half the fun out of eating out. So I walk in and go through my usual spiel with the manager.

"Are you familiar with gluten?" (Blank stare...not a good sign.)

"Is the sushi rice cooked with soy sauce or just vinegar?"

"Any chance of cross-contamination in the kitchen?"

Blah, blah, blah, blah...

It all seems safe. So I order my usual dish: three salmon and avocado rolls. I ask for the spicy mayo sauce on the side and again ask about the sauce to make sure it is ok. I am assured it is.

We eat. We enjoy.

As I take my last bite, the manager comes over and informs us there's been a mistake. The spicy mayo sauce does have gluten in it. Our jaws hit the floor. "You're telling me now??????"

> 2017 Gluten Dude: This was my last spicy mayo ever. Now I enjoy my sushi more than ever with NO SAUCE of any kind, even gluten-free soy sauce. You actually taste...the sushi. Go figure.

Guess what the manager did next? Let's play multiple choice. Did the manager:

a) Give us the check, charging us full price for both of our meals?
b) Charge me a dollar extra for my poisoned sauce?
c) Both of the above?

If you guessed C, pat yourself on the back.

Now this is the first time I had ever known that I had gotten glutened so I had no idea what to expect. Would I start projectile vomiting on the table? Would I die a slow, tortuous death? Would I spend the next 5 days in the bathroom?

So what happened? Well, at first...nothing. That night...nothing. The next day...nothing. Was my GI doctor wrong? Maybe I don't have celiac and it's all been a big mistake.

And then on the second day...BAM! Like a ton of gluten-free bricks. Pure exhaustion. Stomach pains. Anxious. Just a mess. I was a physical and emotional wreck. Lack of focus. Lack of patience. Couldn't sleep enough. And it lasted for SIX MONTHS. Wouldn't wish it on my worst enemy.

So if you have celiac and you're tempted to just have a little gluten, please don't. And if you're in Langhorne PA looking for sushi...well...don't say I didn't warn you.

We are the 1%!

With celiac disease affecting just a little less than 1% of the population, I think it's time to give a little love and attention to our plight. We are not asking for pity...just a bit of an understanding of what us celiacs go thru on a daily basis.

We are the 1% who:

- Must look up ingredients online to see if a product is gluten-free each and every time we are offered something new to eat.

- Spend about three times as much money on gluten-free groceries.

- Have to give a speech to the server every time we go out to eat (and still worry the entire meal).

We are the 1% who:

- Sing Happy Birthday, but don't celebrate with a piece of cake.

- Order the same thing at our favorite restaurant every time we go, because we know it's "safe".

- Must eat our gluten-free rice pasta in one day, because the next day it's as hard as a rock.

We are the 1% who:

- Don't feel well and wonder "Did I get glutened or am I just sick?"

- Begin to forget words, names and dates and realize "Yep, I was glutened."

- Must go back to our previous 9 meals and figure out how we got glutened.

We are the 1% who:

- Usually give up dairy as well.

- Usually give up soy as well.

- Wonder "What the hell *can* I eat?"

We are the 1% who:

- Go to an "all-you-can-eat" buffet, which quickly turns into a "I'll-watch-everyone-else-eat" buffet.

- Miss our occasional Sunday brunch of french toast or pancakes.

- Long for the day of spontaneous living.

We are the 1% who:

- See a bread crumb in our gluten-soy-dairy free butter (yum!) and wonder "Is that a Canyon Bakehouse crumb or did one of my kids just contaminate it?"

- Watch our daughter put her hand in the ice cube tray while eating a bagel.

- Observe a helpful guest wash our gluten-free pots with the wrong-colored sponge.

We are the 1% who:

- Just don't feel "right" a lot of the time.

- Hate complaining about it.

- Wish there were a cure for celiac disease.

Now get on out there a hug a celiac today!

Celiac and the Link to Other Diseases

2017 Gluten Dude: This has been one of the most-read articles on my blog. It has garnished tens of thousands of views and 358 comments, which I suggest you read, as people continue to share THEIR health stories. It's crazy how much I learn from the people who leave comments. Crazy I tell ya!!

I have celiac disease. This fact is pretty well-known by this time. But I haven't shared my other health issues with you. Heck...even the Dudettes (my kids) don't know the whole story. Thankfully, they could care less about my blog so they won't find out.

The reason that I am baring my soul (so to speak) is that I'm curious if there is a connection between celiac disease and the many other health issues I've encountered. I figure if I share my story, perhaps I can entice you folks to do the same and we can do some kind of unscientific study. If I win a Nobel, I will be sure to share the glory.

So here is a list of the health issues I've dealt with:

- In my youth (ages 8-14), I had **WARTS**. Some on my knee. Some on my hands. Not disfiguring mind you. Just annoying. Eventually, they went away.

- At age 10, I woke up one day not feeling well. We had a doctor who lived down the street come by and he suggested I get to the hospital right away. (To this day, I am wondering what he saw in me that made him suggest that. I felt like I just had a cold.) Anyway, I spent 7 long days in the hospital. Blood work out the kazoo. Diagnosis: unknown. I found out years later that they were testing me for **RHEUMATOID ARTHRITIS**. By the way, the highlight of the week was my dad visiting my every night after work and we'd watch *Hogan's Heroes* together. It's funny the things you remember.

- In my teen years, I had the pleasure of dealing with **ACNE**. Worse than many; not as bad as some.

- *At this point, I know what you're thinking. "Wow…warts AND acne. You must have been quite the catch." Yeah…good times indeed.*

- Fast forward to my late twenties and I developed **LOWER BACK PAIN**. Severe at times. It's something I still deal with and actually am currently in physical therapy for it.

- In Spring 2007, I began peeing blood. Diagnosis: **BLADDER CANCER**. And you males out there don't want to know how they diagnose it. Uh…huh. It was low-grade and after one reoccurrence, I've been cancer free (phew!!).

- In Spring 2008, after years of complaining of stomach aches and losing 15 pounds, I finally listened to Mrs. Dude and went to a GI. Diagnosis: **CELIAC DISEASE**.

- In Fall 2008, working one night, starting feeling "not right". Pain in my neck and shoulder…hurt to inhale. Mrs. Dude said we should go to hospital. Do you think I learned my lesson? Of course not. Lying in bed, had a strange sensation. Almost like back pain, but in my entire torso. Jumped out of bed. Feeling went away. Mrs. Dude spent the entire night poking me in the back to make sure I was alive. The next day, my doc said I should go to emergency room just to get it checked out. After five hours of tests, diagnosis: **MULTIPLE BLOOD CLOTS IN BOTH OF MY LUNGS** (medical term: pulmonary embolism). That strange sensation I had was the clots passing thru my heart into my lungs. This is the point in time where most people die from this. Seriously…WTF!?

2017 Gluten Dude: Last month I was both crapping and peeing blood. Had an Endoscopy. Cystoscopy. Colonoscopy. Ran out of "oscopy" tests. Nothing found. Never a dull celiac moment.

So that's my story. Are they related? I have no idea. But I'm thinking there has got to be something going on that ties at least some of it together. I'd love to hear your stories.

Cheating On Your Gluten-Free Diet? Keep it to Yourself.

You're too weak and you wanna cheat on your gluten-free diet? Go for it. It's your early funeral. I just have one simple request.

KEEP IT TO YOURSELF AND DON'T DO IT IN PUBLIC!

When you've got celiac disease, I'm a big believer that you represent the celiac community. And with that comes a responsibility to our community. And if you knowingly cheat, you are making it more difficult for the rest of us to be taken seriously.

I see it on Twitter time and again; celiacs who think they are being cute when they're really being idiots. Stuff like this:

"Ooops…I shouldn't have that bagel but it looked soooo good. I'm so bad. #celiac"

"I am so going to regret having that piece of pizza. #celiac"

After seeing these types of posts far too often, I finally spoke up. Here's how a recent Twitter conversation went.

Her: I'm going to start following my gluten-free diet. Celiac disease will never take me. Holy shit are those bagels?

Me: Please don't make it seem like cheating is an option for celiacs. Makes it harder for the rest of us. Thanks.

Her: I'm a celiac and I cheat. I'm not saying everyone has to. It's an option. Anything can give you cancer, it's just a matter of what triggers it. In my case it'll be something I love ((pizza)). Also celiacs is relatively new; people have lived entire lives having it untreated and die from unrelated causes.

Me: I don't care what you do to yourself. All I'm asking is not to publicize it, cause it diminishes the disease. Thanks.

I was trying to keep it civil, while helping her and the community at the same time. Naturally, other boneheads had to jump in and go in attack mode, telling me I was berating this person and being totally condescending. I even got railed on by a fellow celiac, who isn't shy about how much she detests me. Whatever. Social media at its worst.

Look…I personally don't understand anyone who has celiac disease and cheats. It's poison to your body. And a piece of pizza is worth it? I'm not saying the struggle isn't real. I'm not saying the diagnosis isn't absolutely overwhelming at first. And I'm not saying that temptation won't rear its ugly head once in a while.

But do you really want to deal with the following:

"If celiac disease is left untreated, complications ranging from iron deficiency to osteoporosis to cancer may develop. Some of these problems can occur because of the small intestine's reduced ability to digest food and absorb nutrients properly. Other problems may develop from damage to the intestinal lining that may or may not cause noticeable symptoms." – WebMD

As I said, your body…your life.

But celiac disease is the real deal. It sucks and it's life-long. And by your cheating and being public about it, it tells the world that it's ok for celiacs to cheat. It tells the restaurant workers that a little gluten may be ok. And it tells the community that "we" are the ones being too careful.

Be cool. Don't cheat. The life you save may be your own.

And if you do…

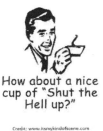

How about a nice cup of "Shut the Hell up?"

My Daddy has Celiac Disease

2017 Gluten Dude: This same Dudette is now in college. Time flies when you can't eat gluten.

Today's special guest blogger is none other than one of the Dudettes...my 13 year old daughter. Mrs. Dude suggested she write a post and I thought the idea was pretty cool. And since it freed me from a day of blogging, I jumped at the opportunity. So what's it like when your dad has celiac disease? Read on to find out.

"

From a kid's perspective, nothing is worse than seeing your parents upset. For me specifically, seeing my dad stand in front of the fridge, not knowing what to eat is the worst. You want to help him and cure everything, but come on, really? A cure? There's no way.

So there he is, standing in front of the fridge, staring. I glance onto the gluten-free shelf, and I see five things, at the most. Most people would start whining (me) and complaining that their life sucks. Not him.

He doesn't complain that he can't eat most food out there. He doesn't complain on family pizza night, when we are enjoying nice cheesy pizza and he is sitting there eating chicken.

He just doesn't. I don't know how he does it, but he does. So what is it like living with a Celiac daddy, you may ask?

Well, when it comes to being active and playing outside, Celiac (for the most part) doesn't come into play. For that, I am very fortunate. My dad did not stop his active life because of this disease. He did not let Celiac ruin his life and how he did it leaves me speechless. So for this, I'm incredibly fortunate.

Then there's the food part. The part where he can't eat what we are eating. Now, I should just say it right off the bat that I am NOT gluten-free. Although I have tried to take a week, I find it literally impossible. No pizza? No bread? Oh my god...NO BAGELS?

I didn't last a day.

But don't let this trick you. Don't be fooled into thinking I don't care. Because believe me, that isn't the case. I think the fact that I couldn't go gluten-free boosted my respect for my dad. Here is he eating 100% gluten-free and I'm sitting next to him eating a bagel. Oops.

Anyway...

The worst part is the guilt. When he gets glutened, you never know what caused it. Was it that new restaurant we went to on Friday? Did the ketchup have hidden gluten in it? Or was it my glutened hand touching the ice. We don't know. You can't blame me for feeling terrible. I just put my dad in two months of misery and there is nothing I can do. Ugh. Celiac sucks. Level of respect for my dad just boosted 100%.

Altogether, I am just extremely grateful that I have a dad who cares so much about the gluten-free community and his health. He is truly inspiring and without a doubt, my role model. I don't know what I would do without him, really. He brightens my mood every day with his charismatic personality. He never fails to make me smile, despite his rough disease.

Celiac has made quite a few bumps in the road. It is not been easy, nor has it been fun. Yet each day he wakes up, ready to start over. He is ready to make a change in the gluten-free world.

My dad believes that his blog is small and not many people follow it.

What he doesn't know is that he is changing lives. Newly diagnosed Celiacs are looking for a voice to guide them; a voice to lead them on the right track. As soon as they find him, they have begun on the road to recovery.

Daddy...you are incredible and you amaze me every day.

You mean the absolute world to me. Stay strong and keep on going. I love you daddy.

I can't even say that enough. I love you.

"

Dear Gluten

2017 Gluten Dude: I had a small contest a few years back. PF Chang's sent me a $100 gift card. I wasn't going to use it (you'll see why in a later chapter), so I wanted to give it away to a fellow celiac. So I asked the community to write a letter to gluten. In other words, what would they say to gluten if given the chance? And then I'd pick a random winner from the bunch. Here are a few that stand out. Enjoy.

Dear Gluten,
I do not knead you anymore.
Love Theresa

————

Dear Gluten,
I hate you. The end.
Hatefully yours,
Amanda

————

Dear Gluten,

I already told you, it's over. I don't know why you have to show up everywhere I go. I go to a birthday party, there you are in the cake, as if that is supposed to tempt me. You show up in breads delivered in the restaurant. You should know better-that is far too obvious. Sometimes you try to sneak into bean dip, even, but I am watching you.

At our company banquet you thought you'd sneak by my lips through omission of information about the menu. Fat chance, I anticipated your move and skipped out. I wasn't about to let you embarrass me. I would have been sick for weeks if I had let that happen.

It's not going to work. I've got rice and tapioca and corn now, and they treat me so much better. They can hide in cake too, and they make it pretty delicious and they make me feel so good. Even my other friends want them. You should be jealous because pretty soon no one is going to want you and your fake genes. Everybody knows by now that a big part of you has been enhanced. Genetic modification is never the answer.

It's over-get over it. I'm not coming back. EVER.

Carrie

_____

Dear Gluten,

You are such a jerk! You have ruined some of my favorite foods! You have to stop crashing my parties and dinners you stalker! Every time you show up, the "silly ass disease" comes with you! I have had to make new friends and try new things. Not everything works out but I keep trying and trying. Not everyone understands why I have to be so careful about you popping up but they try to be understanding. So goodbye Gluten, be a stranger and don't let the door hit you in the silly ass on your way out!

Dana

_____

Dear Gluten,
I miss you. You make bread and cakes so happy and fluffy. You also make my stomach bloated and unhappy but that's ok because it tastes so delicious.

You sly trickster you. You tease me with your delicious fluffiness when I can't have you. Celiac says you make me sick. If it came down to it, you know it would be you I pick.

But now I am Gluten Free. Interesting how much better it can be. So If one more thing can be said. I would like to say that I'd take rice or corn instead.

Sincerely,
Tricia

———

Dear Gluten,

I am 21, and never had a real beer. I will always get drunk faster than my friends because I can only drink hard liquor. I will never play beer pong or flip cup. I will never do a keg stand. I will always be broke because my drinks cost way more than a $5 pitcher.

No more late night Waffle House runs. No more ordering pizza at 5am. No more living off Ramen noodles and Pop Tarts.

Thank you, Gluten, for making my college experience utterly unique.

Sincerely,
The Healthiest College Student Ever

———

Dear Gluten:

When we broke up, I was 44 years old. I had had decades of pizza, cakes, flour tortillas, etc. But, why oh why, do you have to target the kids. Why do you ruin every child's class pizza party, every child's birthday party, and even the college rights of passage – beer!

I don't even miss you anymore. You are toxic to me!

Donna in Denver

———

Dear Gluten,

Once, you were my best friend. You were there to comfort me in times of stress, and to celebrate my victories.

Then, the symphony began. The gastric distress you caused has been endemic. Friends refer to the cacophony of sounds that your gas has invoked.

I became aware that you and I needed to part company. Oh sure, the scale thanked me and my food bills increased, while my stomach settled down. Vanity was not part of the equation. Being healthy, without the gastric distress you caused, feels better than any joy you ever brought me.

Farewell Gluten, hello healthy!

———

Dear Gluten,

You do not define me.

It's been a roller coaster of emotions since you packed your bags and left my intestines 9 years ago. You thought you were cool and all that..partying it up.. wreaking havoc on my villi. It was good to rid of you…but I do digress from time to time with the sweet memories of convenience that you provided me. It's ok. I'm ok. I'm actually better than ok. Since you've been gone, my life has changed for the better. It's true, you did a lot of damage for 33 years and I suffer from that. But I choose the bright side. My glass is half full and you can't take that from me, Mister. I am happy to have my feet firmly planted on the earth instead of beyond. Because a gluten-free life can be a really good life. Your absence has allowed me to meet new people and explore different possibilities. That part is awesome. I know you miss me and lurk around every corner. It's sly of you to try and slip back in once in a while. Such is life. You do not define me, gluten.

"I" define me.

―――

Dear Gluten,
You are such a sneaky little booger. Just when I think I've gotten rid of you, I find out about another place you're showing up. When will you get the hint and stay out of my life and the products I need & want.

―――

Dear gluten,

I am just writing to say that I am soooo over you. I thought the breakup would be hard but I am the happiest I have ever been. I was so tired of being dragged down by you! Thanks for making it so easy to get over you.

Ps- the least you can do is make your presence blatantly apparent instead of sneaking into things! I wish you were neon green so I would at least know when you were around.

―――

Dear gluten,
Shall i compare thee to a tempting thing
thou art more sneaky and more damaging
Rough days do taunt me with your tempting smell,
And restaurant's hath all too small a choice
Sometime too much the tears stream from my face
And often is your good dimmed by the pain
And every bread and treat will lose their awe,
Whole Foods will make the troubles fade away
But my fear of you grows with every day
And just a speck of crumb on my fresh plate
Will leave me with a pain won't go away
When in the past i ate you every day
I now eat free from your long lasting ways
So long live I and this gives hate to thee.

(a parody of Shakespeare's Sonnet 18)

-Annabelle

———

Gluten Rap
You never cease to amaze me,
How you look so good and then play me.
You always keep it together, make things rise,
Then I feel the betrayal deep inside.
So tasty, so smooth, but I gotta get rid –
Gotta find a new base to my pyramid.
Everywhere I look, there you are – so sly
The plural of villain – that's what you are to my villi.

———

Dear Gluten (Sung to the tune of Dear Prudence)

Dear Gluten, won't you get out my way?

Dear Gluten, out of my life you'll stay
I've wizened up, I'm through with you
Barley, Malt and Rye grains too
Dear Gluten, won't you get out my way?

Dear Gluten, I finally realized
Dear Gluten, fog lifted from my eyes
My rash is gone, my joints now spring
You muddled up most everything
Dear Gluten, I finally realized

Doctors give run a round
(Round, round, round, round ,round
Round, round, round, round, round)

AhhhhAhhhAhhhAhhh

Dear Gluten, you're going in the trash pile
Dear Gluten, by you I'm not beguiled
My energy I will regain
So in my house you can't remain

Dear Gluten, you're going into the trash pile

Dear Gluten, out of my life you'll stay
Dear Gluten it's a brand new way
I've wizened up, I'm through with you
Barley, Malt and Rye grains too

Dear Gluten, won't you get out my way?

_____

Dear Gluten,

You are bread to me.

-Caitlyn

_____

Dear Gluten,

You make me sick to my stomach. I used to miss you, but since you left my life almost 10 years ago, I'm the happiest and healthiest I've ever been.

My life is so much better without you.

-Jenny

_____

Dear Gluten,

You're such a pest! Sometimes I can have you and you treat me well. Other times, you wanna sneak up on me and ruin my night out with friends. I told you it was over. I told you that I didn't love you anymore. It's all take and no give with you!

I really need you to take this seriously. You'll always be a part of my life-you're everywhere I go. I can't go a day without seeing you, hearing your name or feeling your aftereffects. I wish I could love you, but I just can't and it's time that I do something for myself.

Please understand. You're delicious, but I can't go on like this.

It's me, not you,
Jenn

———

Dear Gluten,

I'm sorry, but we cannot be friends anymore. I love you, but I can tell that you do not feel the same way about me. This one-way relationship just isn't working out anymore. I cannot stand feeling this way.

We must part ways. I will miss you.

Love,
Jacqueline

———

Dear Gluten,

You are the ultimate food tempter. I see you mocking me from the grocery store aisles, I smell you drifting from the bakeries, I can feel your evil presence when I close my eyes. Cakes, cookies, donuts, biscotti's, tarts, quiches, bread, fried foods, you invade everything.

But you are not the only way to satisfy a carb craving. Rice, tapioca, teff, sorghum and more are my defense against you, and as mighty a defense as a girl could want.

So keep trying, gluten. But you're simply not good enough to crush my fortification.

Sincerely,
No Longer Your Plaything

Celiac Disease: Is This as Good as it Gets?

> 2017 Gluten Dude: Another post from when I was still eating "gluten-free" and feeling the effects of it. Dang…I wish I knew 2017 Gluten Dude back back then. 2012 Gluten Dude was pretty clueless. And to be clear, since I've overhauled my diet, I rarely have long bad "celiac stretches" anymore.

A month or so ago, I was in the midst of a pretty crappy stretch health-wise and went all-out to find a cause and a solution for my health woes.

Truthfully, it's been up and down since my diagnosis in 2007 and I simply just wanted to feel "good".

In addition to going to a number of doctors, getting multiple tests and spending a boatload of money, I received a lot of awesome advice from the gluten-free community with a multitude of suggestions. To all of you, I am grateful.

But among all of the suggestions was an email from "Monica" (not her real name) that offered a completely opposite viewpoint; namely that we have celiac and feeling shitty is just the way it's going to be at times. The email was so well-written and really struck a chord with me.

Please read it below and let me know what you think.

Should I stop trying to find the holy grail and accept my health as it is?

Is this simply as good as it gets??

❝

Hey there Gluten Dude….

I wanted to write something on your blog post today about your test results — but as I appear to be of the minority opinion... I don't really want to hear again that I should be continuing to test. I tried to express my opinion about this once before — but while I know everyone is just trying to be helpful....I just don't need to hear it again. So, I will offer you my opinion here.

I am absolutely of the opinion that we have Celiac Disease ...it is here to stay... and this is the way we're going to feel. Period. I have gone through a multitude of tests as well.... all kinds of blood work and scans and have seen multiple "specialists" (but, no there are no Celiac specialists near me.)

They did end up finding a thyroid issue — which I thought I could blame 'all' my issues on, but no. The doc told me I didn't even need to be on the thyroid medication anymore unless I try to get pregnant (which is a whole different topic) because it was such a 'slight' issue. Apparently it was just temporary thyroiditis and while it 'may' flare up again — it wasn't going to be too much of an ongoing issue. I literally cried in my doctor's office when she said that wasn't my problem — because I was banking on that being 'THE' problem that I was going to be able to fix. [sigh!] I even had to endure a 5-hour barium swallow x-ray procedure once. Hey, I figured — I can deal with this as long as they find 'something'. But, again — there was nothing to find.

Sure, I've been told to take probiotics....and I've been told to take vitamins. Yep — been there, done that ....don't feel any different.

So, in all honesty — Dude, I'm done looking. I made that decision about 5 years ago and I'm happier for it. I still have stomach issues of some sort nearly every day (bloating, cramping, etc.) — but I deal with it. I am still tired....but I work around it.

I have just learned to accept that this is who I am — with Celiac.

Now, I see that people are questioning your & Mrs. Dude's kitchen — but i would venture a guess that you guys are pretty damn careful when it comes to your glutenous surroundings. So am I – and I am 99.9% sure I am not getting accidentally glutened. I have been doing this for 10 years – I know when I've gotten glutened and when I haven't. Plus, I must have healed so well on the gluten-free diet initially – that my 2nd doctor couldn't even confirm I ever had Celiac in the first place (without reading the pathology reports from the first biopsy). And, I still feel way better than I did at that point.

Sure, I could give up soy, eggs, all grains…etc., etc…. but my stint with taking dairy out of my diet – was for nothing. So, I would rather ENJOY my food and feel … well, like a person with Celiac …. than eat bird food – and still feel like $%^#. I want to enjoy life as much as possible….. so, this is what I've decided to do.

I have also received the same response from doctors – wow, you're only 35 and your medical chart looks like you're an 80 year old woman. ;- They threw so many drugs at me trying to 'fix me' – it was ridiculous. About 2 years ago, I decided to stop taking 'all' medications – and you know what… I feel exactly the same as I did while taking the medications – if not better.

I also realize that since I was in a crappy marriage at the time… I kept thinking that if I fixed my health problems, the marital problems would be fixed as well. So, I put a LOT of stock into "fixing" myself. So – when there didn't appear to be anything further wrong with me – other than Celiac – then, I realized the problem may lay elsewhere.

I finally moved on from that marriage and I am very happy now with my new husband. I have the exact same symptoms now as I did back then – but I can "live life" with them better now that everything else has fallen into place. It seems like you and Mrs. Dude and the Dudettes have a pretty happy life right now – other than your health issues. I guess what I'm saying is….. even though I am on my 8th week of lying in bed with my back problem…. I STILL say – "It can always be worse".

Put your extra thoughts into your beautiful children (since some of us don't seem lucky enough to have them….) and less into "what's wrong with me".

As far as I see it – there is nothing wrong with you, Dude. You're a happy, healthy (relatively!!), thriving, popular & successful Dude…. with a loving family and supportive friends. Can't ask for much more than that.

So sorry this has gotten so long but back to the topic at hand. I am sure all the Celiac specialists out there would say keep testing, keep testing, keep testing…. but, what if there is nothing to find – and all you end up being is a human pin cushion?? I just don't know if it's true that "if you're eating a gluten-free diet – you're as normal as anyone else". Seriously??

Instead of trying to be a normal person's "normal" – I have decided to live with what appears to be "normal" for me. An important lesson I learned from my previous marriages is that I need to stop being something I am not…. trying to be what someone else wants me to be – I just need to be ME. The right people will love me for who I am (Celiac and all).

I am not necessarily saying quit all testing immediately – you have gone this far, you 'may' want to investigate one or all of the specialists that your doctor recommended – but, at the end of that (which I am also assuming will all turn out 'normal') …. you may want to decide for yourself what I already have – this is me…this is life…. now, I'm just going to live it.

I wish you well – and I wish I could say ….there is a "normal" life out there beyond the rainbow and to just keep striving for it – but I truly believe this is ….as good as it gets

"

A Weak Moment: How Hunger Clouded My Judgement

I read the books on staying healthy. I subscribe to Men's Health. I follow the "healthy living" blogs. And they all say the same thing: Do not let yourself get too hungry. This is when eating mistakes happen (i.e. overeating, eating crap, etc.).

For celiacs, I'd say it's even more problematic. And when we don't have a contingency plan, bad things can happen.

I was invited to a golf outing for charity on Monday about 20 minutes from the Dude Ranch. I had to leave the house at 11:00 and I figured I'd be home by 5 at the latest.

I ate a big breakfast and on the way to the course, I stopped at our local health food store and picked up a variety of four gluten-free bars. I figured I'd eat two on the front nine and two on the back nine and that would hold me over just fine until I got home for dinner.

The weather was perfect and the golf was anything but. My day was a success. I ate my four bars along with about three gallons of water (yeah…it was pretty dang hot outside.)

There was a banquet dinner after the golf but since I knew I couldn't eat there, I figured I'd just pass and have dinner at home.

What I didn't realize is that the banquet dinner was part of the charity. There would be a raffle and a silent auction. And because I was an invited guest, I felt it would have been quite rude to just golf and leave, so I decided to stay.

It was the right thing to do, but my lack of planning cost me.

The banquet lasted a full three hours. By the second hour, I was absolutely starving and I decided to take a peek at the food that was available. It was one of those banquet setups where you served yourself so I waited until all 150 people had gotten their food.

It wasn't pretty.

Pasta…no.

Roast beef prepared with a seasoning…no.

Fish, turkey, right on down the line…no, no, no.

But then I saw fresh, steamed veggies. I knew I shouldn't even think about it but I was beyond hungry. I asked the waiter and he checked with the kitchen. Seasoned with salt and pepper. That's it.

But what about cross-contamination? How was it prepared in the kitchen? Did they use separate utensils?

I didn't ask.

The question is…why didn't I ask?

Was it because I knew they wouldn't have an answer? Or was it because I didn't want to know the answer?

I ate the veggies.

It was risky. It was stupid. It was weak. The ironic thing is I couldn't even enjoy them because I knew I shouldn't be eating them. For 5+ years, I can count on one hand the times I ate something where I knew there was a small risk involved.

And each time, I say never again…it's just not worth it.

But then I have an occasion where I don't plan ahead enough and hunger takes over.

The lesson learned? Always pack more food than you think you need. Always.

The second lesson? Don't beat yourself up over it.

We're only human.

You're Not Crazy. You May Just Have Celiac Disease.

We all know that celiac disease continues to be misdiagnosed and that the average time to get accurately diagnosed is 6-10 years.

We all know that because there is no "cure" for celiac disease and no drugs to treat it, and therefore no financial incentive for the medical community, it often gets overlooked.

What you may not know is that so many people, while trying to find a reason for their ailments, are diagnosed as having psychological issues. Imagine that? A doctor saying you need psychological help simply because he/she can't find a physical reason for all your symptoms.

I hear it over and over again and it frustrates me to my core.

I want share a story that a fellow celiac sent to me. Not only is she a celiac, but she is a registered nurse. And yes…she was told she was crazy.

"

I am a registered nurse and I knew um, nothing about celiac disease prior to my diagnosis. I have worked in the ER for years and yet knew nothing about it!

As a patient, like all celiac sufferers, I have a horrendous story to my diagnosis, but the long and short of it being that although psychiatric problems were the first/second/third thing every GP I've ever been to about the symptoms ever said (it was always in there somewhere), someone finally listened to me and tested the right thing.

I am honestly not surprised about the lack of health community knowledge about celiac, because a) it's not immediately life threatening and b) aren't we (celiac sufferers) all crazy anyways??

I wish I had known something about it, because hell, I would have picked it up myself a lot earlier than anyone else did. As a health professional, I thought I was going crazy with my constant symptoms with no obvious clinical basis, so I just told myself that I was ok and I would just have to live with the constant pain, nausea, diarrhea, vomiting, constipation, teeth problems, nerve problems, etc… list goes on.

Crazy aye, I think I drove myself there, I had no answers so I just ignored it, but it wasn't going away.

My celiac demanded attention and finally I returned to the GP and she mentioned celiac although her third suggestion was maybe I should see the psychologist!! My blood test and biopsies were positive+++ and here I am newly minted gluten-free lifestyle, HEALING!

What I want to know is if it is so common, why aren't GP's encouraged to test those who have iron deficiency and symptoms of leaky gut or vague autoimmune symptoms for it? Why isn't there a bigger push to get them to take notice? Why do we all have to go through so much trauma to get anywhere, anywhere at all with our doctors? How can they diagnose IBS without a clean celiac blood screen? What gives them the right to make us think we are going mad?

Do you know how severely deranged your mental state has to be to be causing actual bodily upset like gastrointestinal symptoms and the others? It has to be pretty high on the level of derangedness!

So turns out I'm not crazy, and I tell myself every day that I am healing now! I am my own health advocate, I am the only person going to look after myself and that is what I am doing now.

Do not rely on your GP; if something is wrong with you, you need to make them understand. It is not in their nature to push past the initial diagnosis to look for something more sinister or hidden unless there are great big arrows pointing them that way. So make those arrows bloody big!

Life goes on. Better and better.

"

I'm So Sorry Our Disease is Such an Inconvenience For You

It never ends. It seriously never ends. The constant ignorance out there and the constant need to defend ourselves about our disease and other food intolerances.

What set me off this time? An utterly ridiculous article on Huff Post titled *"Why Do Your Kid's Allergies Mean My Kid Can't Have a Birthday?"* written by one Carina Hoskisson (Search for it online if you wish. Trust me…it'll turn your stomach.)

It's time for a Gluten Dude breakdown.

Let's start with the title: Right away we have an entitled mom who thinks her child having a piece of birthday cake in school is more important than another child's health. And who's saying your kid can't have a birthday? Won't you celebrate at home? Isn't one cake party enough for him?

She says: *All over the country parents are being asked to accommodate the specialized needs of other people's children thanks to the skyrocketing number of food allergies and food intolerances.*

Dude says: And I wonder why this is. Could it be that half the things many of our kids are eating don't even classify as food? Have you read the ingredients of some of the things out there?

She says: *We can't bring in homemade cookies or snacks; we're asked to buy commercially prepared goods. Even if you agree to bring in commercially prepared snacks, you're asked to make sure they're "gluten, nut, and egg-free" or some other combination of scary food exorcism.*

Dude says: People with allergies can die from one bite. People with celiac disease have their intestines attacked by their own body with one bite. Your kid getting a cupcake is worth this risk to other kids? Really?? Tell me…what color is the sky in your world?

She says: *To a certain extent, I get it. When I was in high school, a girl in my town died from eating a few bites of a Twix bar that happened to contain traces of peanuts.*

Dude says: "To a certain extent" you get it? Someone died and you only get it "to a certain extent"?? No that IS the extent. That's why it's so damn important.

She says: *I would never endanger the life of a child over a peanut butter cookie; that would be ridiculous.*

Dude says: Then what's the point of your article? Let's move on.

She says: *However, I am rapidly reaching the end of my rope. One mom told me there were so many allergies in her children's classes last year that all she could bring was gummy bears and juice boxes. Let me get this straight: I'm supposed to feed my kids processed, preservative-laden food because your kid has a wheat allergy?*

Dude says: In a perfect world, we'd do away with the food parties altogether. It's an old-school tradition that does not seem to have a place anymore. But if the teachers are insistent on having a food party and if processed crap is the only option to keep a kid safe (which we all know it's not), then yeah, you do it.

Again, I ask…why is your child getting a piece of cake more important than another child's health?

She says: *I understand the problem with allergies because I have allergies; I'm allergic to egg whites. The difference is I don't demand egg-free items when I go to parties or to work events.*

Dude says: YOU'RE AN ADULT. You have the willpower to say no. As strong as a celiac child may be, it may be tough if everyone is having a cupcake and he/she feels left out. There is temptation that a child may not have the strength to overcome.

Comparing yourself to a child is ridiculous. Actually, in this case, maybe it's not.

She says: *I agree that a teacher should let all parents know about any life-threatening allergies in a classroom. However, my kid shouldn't have to forgo his birthday cake because yours can't eat it.*

Dude says: Or you can teach your kid a lesson on empathy and tell him *"another child's health is more important than you getting a piece of cake at school…but hey don't worry…we'll have some awesome cake tonight."* Is that so hard to do?

She says: *Some schools have even gone the route of banning all classroom birthdays and celebrations, which is ridiculous.*

Dude says: No, actually…it's not ridiculous. What's ridiculous is that at a time when food allergies are becoming more and more prevalent, there is still such a lack of compassion and understanding. Look…I'm all for balance and I'm all for letting our kids socialize at school and have some fun. But why does it need to be based around food? The only reason is because it's always been done that way. Change takes time. It's time to start.

She says: *Let's stop the allergy insanity, and let the rest of them eat cake — the lovely, homemade, buttery, gluten-stuffed cake.*

Dude says: I have no more words for this woman. I just hope her kids grow up with more tolerance, more empathy and more understanding. Somehow, I doubt it. Cycles are hard to break.

When the Disney fiasco happened and we came together to have them change an episode about gluten-free bullying, the common argument against us was that "this is the pussification of America". It's like they all got the same memo or something. Well, if standing up for something you believe in…if standing up for someone who is portrayed as weak and inferior because he has food allergies…if that's "pussification", then I'm the biggest p***y in the world.

Oh…and here's the topper. As I'm writing this post, some bonehead posted this on Twitter: Kids teacher just emailed saying only gluten-free snacks in the classroom. MY KID DOESNT HAVE CELIAC DISEASE! Ugh, hippies drive me INSANE.

Yep...that's us...just a bunch of hippies with a made up disease.

So sorry for the inconvenience.

A Letter from a Non-Celiac. Wow. Just...Wow.

I know we (or maybe I should say I) complain about the lack of support and understanding from the general population about celiac. I've gotten email after email after email from celiacs who are put through the ringer by those who aren't educated about our disease.

But do you know there is a whole community of non-celiacs out there who have our back? Who understand? Who respect the trials and tribulations we go through?

Check out the email I received recently.

If this doesn't put a smile on your face, you must be seriously botoxed out.

"

Dear Gluten Dude,

This is technically not a rant, but a message I want to share with you and all your fellow celiacs. I know you're busy and have lots of battles to fight and people to educate, so I thank you for taking the time to read my letter. Here it is:

Dear Celiacs,

I understand. I am not a celiac myself, but a dear friend of mine is, so I have spent countless hours researching the topic, adjusting and perfecting my recipes, looking for safe cosmetics that would make a nice birthday present, reading ingredients lists, and reaching out to manufacturers to get information.

And I am not alone. We are committed, and we are many. We are your partners, your friends, your sisters, your brothers, your mothers, your fathers, your sons, your daughters, your aunts, your uncles, your grandparents, your colleagues, your acquaintances, or even complete strangers.

We do our best to spread the word and educate others, so that if they ever come across a celiac, they will treat them with respect and understanding.

We perfect our gluten-free recipes even when we're not cooking for you, so that we can offer you safe, delicious food when you come over. We take action when we find mislabeled products, misleading menus, and inaccurate information.

We care.

So if there ever comes a time when you're feeling desperate, frustrated, misunderstood, all alone in the world, or just plain angry (and with celiac on your plate, how could it not?), think of this letter. Think of us. We are with you always, and we understand.

V.

"

On behalf of the entire celiac community, thank you V. Your words have touched my heart, breathed life into my tired body, and gave me a great reminder of why I advocate so strongly.

I'm pretty speechless…and how often does THAT happen?!

When Celiac Takes Away Your Ability to Carry Your Own Children

Thank god for this blog. Not in a "pat myself on the back" kind of way AT ALL.

But if I didn't start this blog, I would have had absolutely no idea the extent of the havoc celiac plays and how it affects so many people in such a variety of ways. I would have been among the clueless who figured everyone had the same symptoms as me. It has been absolutely eye-opening and I'm beyond grateful people have shared their stories, as hard as some of them are to hear.

The below email comes from Wendy, who had a life-altering conversation with her doctor after her celiac diagnosis. She is not specifically asking for help, but I wanted to share this story just the same. I'm assuming she's not alone in this.

Here's the email...

"

It was after an endoscopy just under 2 years ago that my doctor turned to me and stated, "You need to know that your body cannot sustain a pregnancy right now." As I sat in the doctor's office my throat still slightly sore from the recent procedure, an endoscopy which came after months of unexplained symptoms that worsened to the point my extreme fatigue and weakness caused me to leave my summer job a month early in the hopes of being well enough to face my final year of grad school in a few weeks, I was single and having a baby was far from in my immediate future.

Still at 27 the words and their potential implications for my future stung. The malabsorption from Celiac was wreaking havoc on my

92

body. I could barely keep myself alive, let alone carry a baby at that time.

Now fully committed to a gluten-free lifestyle and much healthier than before, I still hear the doctor's proclamation and wonder if I am now, or will ever be, 'healthy' enough to carry my own children. In addition to Celiac I suffer from an additional currently 'unspecified autoimmune' disorder that is causing me small fiber neuropathy and tremors.

Doctors have told me they really don't know and can't know exactly how my body would react to a pregnancy. I'm in a position I never imagined: 29 and dating and in the back of my mind already knowing that a biological family may not be possible for me.

I wonder when one shares this knowledge with a significant other, if I could marry someone who didn't feel adoption was a choice for them (as adoption is a very real possibility when I think of my future); if I could be okay never having a family of my own.

It is amazing to think that something I ingested multiple times a day for the vast majority of my life would literally eat away at part of me and leave me questioning my future in such major ways.

[Dude note: This line speaks volumes about our disease.]

Whatever happens I know that it will be alright in the end – but I cannot help questioning what it means to know my body may not allow me the choice of carrying my own children…and how I best approach it with those around me.

"

Dermatitis Herpetiformis: The Celiac Rash from Hell

What exactly is dermatitis herpetiformis?

Dermatitis Herpetiformis (DH) is a severe, itchy, blistering skin manifestation of celiac disease that is genetically determined and is not contagious. The name, dermatitis herpetiformis, is a descriptive name and is not related to either dermatitis or herpes, but is a specific chronic skin condition. The rash may occur in the form of small lumps, like insect bites and in some cases form fluid filled blisters. These small blisters are called vesicles. However the rash may appear hive-like, persisting in one area. DH can flare and subside even without treatment. The rash usually occurs on the elbows, knees, and buttocks. When the rash subsides, which it often does spontaneously, it may leave brown pigmentation or pale areas, where pigmentation is lost. (source: celiaccentral.org).

I hear about DH from many in this community but I have never written about it. Kinda one of those things that since I don't have it, I wouldn't know what to say about it. But I got a request from a fellow celiac to please talk about it so we can give those suffering from DH some Gluten Dude love.

And being that her email was so dang cute and persuasive…how could I resist?

So Monika…your itch…I mean your wish is my command.

"

Hey Dude!

You mentioned that May is Celiac Awareness Month, and you're going on your month of helping us in that awesome way that you do. I was hoping I could ask a bit of a favor…*bats eyelashes*

In a recent post, the person who emailed you mentioned having two Celiacs at home with Duhrings disease. I got kind of excited because Duhrings/Dermatitis Herpetiformis is so often forgotten in the Celiac conversation, or at best is usually just an afterthought "oh yea, and you might get a rash…and now back to crapping your pants…"

For some background info…for about 20+ years I got run of the mill diagnoses of eczema/dermatitis, and we never thought much of it. As a kid, my mom get special soaps, creams, fancy bath stuff, plain cotton clothing…and I just dealt with my ever worsening itching and pain. I'd have these awful reactions and not be able to function. I'd be freaking out with an anxiety attack, crying over my computer trying to handle all the constant work that grad school throws at you while wanting to tear my skin off and die.

I tried researching if this could be something specific, I even tried looking up autoimmune diseases at a friend's suggestion…and I just couldn't find much. I eventually figured out some kind of wheat connection after the awful linguini incident of ought twelve. I sorta ran with that as it was all the information I had to go off of…and I didn't really know what to do with it.

In the way that so much of the population is oblivious to Celiac, I knew nothing of it. I had a coworker a couple years back who had some stomach thing, that's it. It wasn't until my sister started talking about Celiac that I started to figure this out a bit. When my rashes stopped, and I kept researching, I finally found a mention of DH and nearly started crying. I finally found something that described what I had.

It's really fitting for me that May is Celiac Awareness Month, because the end of April marks my one year totally gluten-free anniversary. The amazing year that I finally figured out my DH and immensely improved my quality of life by changing my eating habits. I feel amazing, and I want to shout it from the rooftops.

Here's where that favor from so many paragraphs ago comes in…Dearest Dude, I guess I just wanted to ask you to highlight DH a bit. You've mentioned it in the past and, along with all the work you do, I love you for it. Maybe a tinge more though? I find that most times it isn't even mentioned by name, just as "rash" under other Celiac symptoms.

The best description I've heard is this it's like "rolling in stinging nettles naked with a severe sunburn, then wrapping yourself in a wool blanket filled with ants and fleas…" Which is so much more than "oh yea, you might get a bit itchy."

So far this link has had the most comprehensive information, and it's what I share with people if they ask: http://blog.glutenfreeresourcedirectory.com/dermatitis-herpetiformis-when-celiac-disease-gets-under-your-skin/

So, pretty please with a cherry on top? Do me a favor and give us 15-25% of Celiacs with mutinous skin a bit of the spotlight?

Thanks Dude!!
<3 Monika

You're quite welcome Monika. Happy to get the word out and show some lovin' for those suffering from DH. My heart goes out to you.

"

Gluten Ataxia: When Celiac Messes with Your Brain

So I woke up feeling "celiac off" yesterday. I went to bed feeling really "off" last night. And this morning, I'm feeling so "off", I just put a note outside my home office door that says "please do not disturb".

When I'm feeling this "off", human interaction is not my friend. I'm agitated. I'm irritated. Let's face it…I become an a**hole.

No…I have no idea what happened or what I ate that was the culprit. It's the crap shoot that is our disease. We eat outside of our home, we run a risk. We can mitigate that risk as much as humanly possible, but it's still a risk.

I'm amazed, even after all of these years, how much celiac can affect my entire being when I ingest gluten.

And this is the perfect segue into an email I received recently that deals with Gluten ataxia.

What is gluten ataxia?

Well…ataxia is a lack of muscle coordination which may affect speech, eye movements, the ability to swallow, walking, picking up objects and other voluntary movements. A person with persistent ataxia may have damage in the part of the brain that controls muscle coordination – the cerebellum. (Source: Medical News Today).

Gluten ataxia occurs when the antibodies that are produced in response to the ingestion of gluten attack the cerebellum. Left untreated, the condition progresses, causing irreversible brain damage.

I was not too familiar with gluten ataxia until I received the following email from a fellow celiac:

,,

Hi Gluten Dude,

I am a 29 year old male and I was diagnosed late last year with Celiac Disease and Gluten Ataxia, after what was, the doctor's think, at least 10 years of undiagnosed suffering. Undiagnosed because I was largely asymptomatic until the later stages of the disease. Right around the time I went to college, the first symptoms started to arise in the form of chronic acid reflux and an ever swelling little pot belly.

Despite being a runner, my gut continued to distend and grow over the course of my 20s until my once 5'11" 160 lb runners frame had blown out to nearly 230 lbs. My self-image became pretty well shattered. I was frustrated because of my inability to lose weight despite constant exercise, and attempted dieting (though I was always, always hungry).

Right around 2011, I started dropping into bouts of depression, initiated by a variety of things but largely because despite everything I did I never felt good, I always felt sick. My blood sugar would frequently crash, I was catching mystery illnesses all the time, and the doctors would chalk it up to my obesity and "poor" lifestyle.

In 2014 the symptoms started to go neurological, with frequent dizzy spells, and slow loss of motor control first in my left hand, then the left side of my face and tongue and periodic feeling of drunkenness.

Late last year the Gluten Ataxia blew up, until one night, after a quick dinner and couple beers with friends, I spent the evening on my bathroom floor, unable to swallow, choking on my own spit, unable to control my muscles well enough to do anything but crawl across the floor to the toilet, where I had to let the spit just drool out of my mouth rather than what felt like drowning on it.

I'd had enough then of doctors putting me off. I sat in waiting rooms and demanded that they fix me, and eventually they figured it out. My small intestine was severely damaged and I was holding an inflamed mass of water around my gut. The MRI showed lesions on my cerebellum from the Ataxia, brain damage that will never go away and always make my fine motor control in my left hand difficult.

6 months after the diagnosis, and an extreme diet that also rid me of dairy, I do not remember feeling better in my adult life. I'm crying here as I write this. I dropped 30 lbs of inflammation in a month. Though I'm not as skinny as I was, I'm now a much more manageable 190 lbs. Though my diet is limited, I enjoy food in a way I never did before, now free of reflux, bloating and cramping. I am, by every metric, a happier man.

Thanks for the opportunity to let it all out on paper Gluten Dude.

,,

Crazy, right? Brain damage caused by something we eat.

This disease never ceases to amaze me.

CVS Will No Longer Check My Meds for Gluten. Here's Why.

Have a seat. I'll tell you a story, *The Princess Bride* style. I'll play the role of Peter Falk and you can be Fred Savage. (Hello. My name is Inigo Montoya. You killed my father. Prepare to die.)

About two months ago, I was having a medical issue that shall remain anonymous. I saw my doc and she suggested I take what we'll call Drug X. She gave me a sample and off I went.

Naturally, I had to look up Drug X to see if it was gluten-free because lord knows **OUR MEDICATIONS DO NOT HAVE ANY LABELING LAWS**. So off to glutenfreedrugs.com I went and crap…it wasn't listed. Now that doesn't necessarily mean it's not gluten-free. It's just not on the list. I searched and I searched and finally found one legit medical website that said the Drug X is indeed gluten-free.

So I began to take Drug X. Was there a slight risk it was not gluten-free? I suppose and I'm not one for risks when it comes to celiac, but I felt it was important enough and if it turns out it was NOT gluten-free, I'd know it within a few days.

Well, a few days went by and no reaction. Not only that, but Drug X was working for me. It was relieving my symptoms. So I finished the sample and then put in a prescription at CVS to fill the next month's supply.

When I went to pick up the medication, they said they could not give it to me because it was not gluten-free. It turns out the list they go by is glutenfreedrugs.com. That's the only list they go by. And since it was not on the list, they decided it was not safe for me.

Dude note: Kudos to CVS for the efforts up to this point. Honestly.

Anyway, I said that I found a medical site that said Drug X was gluten-free and also informed them that I've been on it for a month with no ill effects, so I'm ok taking it. They marked it in their system that I was taking the medication against their advice and off I went.

A month later, I went to the doc after not being able to shake whatever virus has been wreaking havoc on my body and soul the past 10 days. My doc prescribed a cough syrup and an antibiotic.

So off to CVS I went to drop off the prescriptions. When I dropped them off, I reminded them to please check for gluten in these medications. They said no…they will not check.

EXCUSE ME??

They said because I took Drug X when they could not confirm it was gluten-free, they will no longer check any of my medications for gluten and they actually wiped celiac off of my charts. The head pharmacist came over and confirmed. In their minds, I no longer have celiac disease and will not be treated as such.

I was absolutely floored. And a day later, I still am.

Perhaps it's a legal thing and they are just covering their asses. Perhaps they have a god complex. Perhaps this one pharmacist was just an **hole. Perhaps I'm missing something here. I have no idea but man, what a shitty way to do business.

And by the way, I still picked up the other two meds but looked them up on my phone before actually purchasing them. One was on "the list" but the cough syrup was not. Here we go again. I purchased them both and did more research at home, with the assistance of Mrs. Dude and Cousin Julie. It was indeed on the list…just under a different name.

We have such a long way to go folks. I've been in conversation with some of my favorite celiacs about banding together to really push for medication labeling laws. Now I'm more motivated than ever.

Anyway…that's my story. Sure, there were no 6-fingered men or rodents of unusual size, but it's the best I've got.

Let's Talk About Poop

Today's topic of discussion
Is simple and clear
We're talking about our bodies
And the stuff that comes out of our rear

I know it's not easy
And it may make you feel a bit loopy
But what is more natural
Than taking a little poopie?

No need to be squeamish
It's not something to miss
As we converse about what happens
When I squeeze a Hershey's Kiss

You see ever since celiac
My deuces have been runny
For all of you in the same boat
You know that this ain't funny

It's been awful, it's been messy
When I go in the dumpy
There is just nothing fun
When I push out a grumpy

Celiac does a number
On my intestinal tract
Out of nowhere I get that feeling
"OMG…I've got to take a crap!"

I run to the bathroom
Or you can call it the pooper
But no matter what you call it
I drop a nasty state trooper

So six years and running
I've taken my lumps
But now things have brightened
When I take my dumps

They're solid, they're clean
Like god meant them to be
Now it's not so bad
Going to the crap factory

So what have I changed?
What have I done?
Why is going number two
Now as easy as going number one?

Let me explain
I'll lay it all out on the table
Why not it's not so unpleasant now
When I lay some cable

Five months ago
I listened to a voice
That said feeling so crappy
Doesn't need to be a choice

I'd already given up dairy
Along with soy and corn
But I needed to do more
And take the bull by the horn

So I hit the pharmacy
CVS to be exact
To purchase some vitamins
That perhaps my body lacked

I brought a Probiotic
Nature's Bounty is the brand

And Vitamin B-complex
To help me in the can

I took them every morning
I didn't miss a day
I wished and prayed and hoped
That my loose doodies would go away

And boy oh boy wouldn't you know it
Within a week I said "See ya"
To all those chocolate squirts
And nasty diarrhea

Now I'm in and out
I don't make a gigantic fuss
Dare I say it's almost enjoyable now
Riding the porcelain bus?

So if you've got some issues
When you're in the loo
Try to do as I did
And see if it helps your poo

Again...that's Probiotics and B-complex
This is my big scoop
I really hope it helps
Next time you take a poop

What Does Celiac Disease Mean to You?

I have a page on my website called *Faces of Celiac Disease* (if you are not on the page, get your mugshot up there). When a fellow celiac submits their picture, I ask them to complete this sentence:

Celiac disease…

They have 75 characters to say what celiac disease means to them. I'd like to highlight a few of the 1400+ answers so far. And since it's my book, that's what I'm going to do. Take note that celiac means so many different things to so many of us. We're all affected by this autoimmune disease in our own personal way.

After reading these, tell me…what does celiac disease mean to you??

- Celiac disease is a serious autoimmune disease.

- Celiac disease is misunderstood.

- Celiac disease is sometimes sad and aggravating but we are GF to stay healthy and happy!

- Celiac disease is a challenge — one that I meet head-on every day (mostly successfully).

- Celiac disease makes me feel very isolated sometimes.

- Celiac disease can't stop me from seeing the world and enjoying life!

- Celiac disease is more than just a change in one's lifestyle.

- Celiac disease is a disease that makes eating a very involved, complicated puzzle.

- Celiac disease attacked my central nervous system and nearly destroyed me before diagnosis.

- Celiac disease has not stopped me from smiling and just being a kid!

- Celiac disease saved my life.

- Celiac disease has given me ups and downs but this is who I am and I've come to accept it.

- Celiac disease nearly killed me. Twenty years on, I'm still trying to live with it.

- Celiac disease means my mommy makes me yummy healthy food. I still get cookies!

- Celiac disease is a pain in the ass but could definitely be worse!

- Celiac disease is NO JOKE! A 100% gf diet saved me from a life of pain and misery.

- Celiac disease heightens my awareness of what I put into my body.

- Celiac disease is annoying! People think that I'm a hypochondriac.

- Celiac disease has forced me to learn how to cook and eat healthier. I now love to cook!

- Celiac disease is a lot of work. But I'm glad to have answers.

- Celiac disease has given me a new appreciation for life.

- Celiac disease makes it difficult for me to feel comfortable going out with my friends.

- Celiac disease is finally the answer to why I have felt like crap for years.

- Celiac Disease is hard for a kid but does not define who I am!

- Celiac disease gives me, uh, what was the question? Oh ya, brain fog!

- Celiac disease was a diagnosis that helped me learn how I could save my own life.

- Celiac disease is what I have, but not who I am.

- Celiac disease has been a curse, but also a blessing, making me eat more healthy.

- Celiac disease has caused distrust in the medical field.

- Celiac disease has made me realize I'm stronger than I thought.

- Celiac disease was an answer to my prayers. I was very ill and just wanted to know why.

- Celiac disease is harder physically, mentally and spiritually then can be put into words.

- Celiac disease does not make me a bad dinner guest.

- Celiac disease is not a fad.

- Celiac disease is a bumpy ride and an epic journey!

- Celiac disease freaking sucks (I thought I'd finish strong)!

As for me, and I am granting myself more than 75 characters, celiac disease is a constant unwanted companion. It never leaves me. And yet, in a perverse kind of way, I am also thankful for it. I control my disease with food. I have made great friends within the community. I have become a "voice"; not one that everyone loves, but still. And this may sound odd, but it has given my life a kind of purpose that I did not have before I launched this blog.

I will ask one simple thing of you today. Try to find one person that you can spread celiac awareness to. That's it. Just one person. Together, we can and will make a difference.

How to Cut Through the Gluten-Free Hype

Gluten-free has become an untamed monster. Whenever there is money to be made, the fad soon follows. And holy-moly has gluten-free become a fad. I just did a search on Amazon for "gluten-free books". Guess how many results it returned. 100? 1,000? How about 20,443! That's insane.

The question becomes…how do you know who to listen to (besides me of course)? With thousands of books, thousands of websites and thousands of opinions, many of them uneducated, how do you cut through the crap and do what's right for you? How do you know who is in it for profit and who is in it for passion?

I get emails from fellow celiacs; lots and lots of emails. Some with heartbreaking stories; some with inspiring stories of success; some with great questions; some with medical questions that I cannot (and will not) answer; and some that just want to say thanks (I love those!)

But I also get my share of emails that go something like this:

- "I heard from [random source] that [random gluten-free food] has gluten in it."

- "I heard from [random source] you can get glutened walking through the flour aisle in the grocery store."

- "I heard from [random source] that eating out is always dangerous."

Although I tend not to answer those types of emails that are either grossly misinformed or fear-based, my responses would be something like this:

"No it doesn't."
"No you can't."
"No it isn't."

Getting the facts straight about celiac disease and gluten-free is so important to those in our community. So let's get some nasty myths out of the way, shall we?

Myth: Coffee contains gluten.
Truth: If it did, I'd be dead. Not sure about flavored coffees, but then again, that's not really coffee. Yes…I'm a coffee snob.

Myth: Hard alcohol is not gluten-free.
Truth: See my coffee answer above.

Myth: A gluten-free diet is unhealthy and should only be followed if you are a celiac.
Truth: Horse-hockey. My diet is plenty healthy. I eat vegetables. I eat fruit. I eat meat. I eat fish.

Myth: You can absorb gluten through your skin and cause a celiac reaction.
Truth: Nope. Dr. Fasano says "it is the oral ingestion of gluten that activates the immunological cascades leading to the autoimmune process typical of celiac disease."

Myth: You will lose weight on a gluten-free diet.
Truth: If you eat cookies, cakes and donuts, gluten-free or not, you ain't losing weight. Not to mention the fact that many celiacs are malnourished when first diagnosed, so odds are you'll gain weight at the beginning as your body heals and begins absorbing nutrients again.

Myth: Gluten-free should mean 0 parts per million, not 20ppm.
Truth: Currently, the best that we can test for is 3ppm. And most researchers agree that 20ppm is the safe threshold for celiacs. While I'd like to see us be more stringent, demanding 0ppm isn't the answer.

Myth: You can get tested and diagnosed with non-celiac gluten-sensitivity.
Truth: There is no valid test for this…yet.

Myth: Taking a gluten-digestion pill before a meal will allow you to eat gluten.

Truth: Don't fall for this baloney and put money in these people's pockets. You cannot eat gluten, no matter what you do.

So who do you trust? (Or if you're George Thorogood, who do you love?) My best recommendation is to follow your gut. And sure…pun intended…why not. I don't want to mention any specific names, but there are a lot of great people out there who are in the business of gluten-free for the right reasons. Find these people. They don't fear-monger. They don't give you a hard sell. They are in the gluten-free community because they have something to offer that comes from a good place.

Who don't you trust? How about the media. So much of the media just sucks. You know that. I know that. Too many of them care only about clicks and ratings and not about truth and consequences. It's the world we live in and it's not gonna change.

Perhaps it would change if people would stop buying trash magazines and stop watching crap Reality TV and showed the world that we are indeed an "educated consumer". But until then, it's "market to the bottom feeders and collect your money."

And now the media has taken on gluten. Full force. Here are some recent headlines from some major publications:

"Gluten-Free Fad Debunked"
"Gluten-Free Health Benefits are Overhyped"
"Gluten-Free Food Isn't Actually Any Healthier for Most of Us"
"Gluten-Free Fad Costing Buyers More with Little Benefit"
"Gluten-Free Food Not Healthier At All"

And to all of those publishers I say this: No duh.

Of course the fad is ridiculous. (The same fad you were more than happy to write all about as long as it brought you click$.)

Of course the gluten-free version of most similar products are no healthier. (But hey, let's all celebrate that there are now 37 varieties of gluten-free chocolate chip cookies on the shelves.)

Of course it's more expensive to buy gluten-free food. (And if you buy naturally gluten-free, even more so.)

The celiac community has been screaming this for years. Well…I've been screaming. I won't speak for the rest of you. And it's not really screaming by definition since I'm writing it, not speaking it. THIS IS SCREAMING. This is talking firmly!! We can move on now.

Heck, even The Huffington Post seems to be writing an article a day about gluten now. You can usually find them right next to their stirring *"Britney Spears doesn't look like THIS anymore!!"* articles. Journalism at its finest.

Here's my hope…and I've been hoping this for some time now: The media just moves on to something else. They can earn their editor's badge on another topic that they will then beat to death. There must be a Kardashian or two that haven't gotten the attention they crave. Gluten has been played out. Give it back to the celiac and NCGS community where it belongs.

As for the rest of you…if eating gluten-free makes you feel better, don't eat gluten. It's really that simple. Don't listen to the media and the crap they serve up. Don't fall for the companies that are strictly in this for profit. Pay no attention to the "sky is falling" people who say gluten is everywhere and you should fear for your health.

It's all about balance. Always has been and always will be.

And one last piece of advice as I wind things down. Listen to your body. It will never steer you wrong.

Chapter 3: Eating RIGHT. Not Just Gluten-Free.

And this is where my journey to better health truly began (and yours will too).

If you are like me, and I'd say 95% of newly diagnosed celiacs, the first thing you did upon your diagnosis was go to the store and empty their shelves of all of the gluten-free food you could find.

Gotta have cookies still.
Gotta have pizza still.
Gotta have bread still.
Gotta have [whatever] still.

Wrong. Wrong. Wrong. If there is only one thing you get out of this book, it's to avoid this mistake. I was sick for years after my diagnosis. Why? I didn't know. I was so beyond frustrated and Mrs. Dude was at her wits end too. Eating "gluten-free" wasn't doing the trick. And forget the fact that I also put on almost 20 pounds. I felt like absolute crap and I knew deep inside that food was the reason. I had to make a change.

First step...I gave up dairy. Not an easy thing to do but I knew it was another top allergen. Definitely made a difference. But not enough of one.

Second step...gave up corn, since it's hard to digest. Made another slight difference but was still hurting.

Finally...I gave up almost all gluten-free food and started eating real food. My first foray into this was doing the Whole30. Absolutely life-changing for me. After 30 days, I lost weight and felt great. There was no turning back.

This is not to say I did not have my off-days and I felt great 100% of the time. That's just the nature of the celiac beast. And yeah…I had a few stretches where I didn't treat my body right. And I paid for it. Every. Single. Time.

And when I was going through a stage of not feeling well, I did the AIP diet and again…just wow…what a difference.

And I haven't bought a box of gluten-free crap since. Do I miss it? Not one bit.

Keep reading to learn more about my journey to "eating right." You won't be sorry. Happy healing!!

Dear Dairy

See what I did there? Instead of Dear Diary, I cleverly inverted the two letters? I know…you don't have to say it.

Dear Dairy,

It's been a great run. When I was a child, my 3 brothers and I would polish off a gallon of you every single day.

I loved you in my homemade tortellini and cream sauce.

Roast beef and provolone sub? My favorite.

And who can forget all the cheeseburgers we shared together.

And those omelets…oh my, don't even get my started.

And finally, for the last few years, we'd start our day together at 5am with our coffee.

But it's time for us to part ways. It's nothing personal, I assure you. It's just that whenever we spend time together, I always end up feeling worse. And when that happens, it's time to end the relationship and move on. You can even ask Dr. Phil.

And one final thing. It's not your fault. It's not your fault. It's not your fault. (Picture Matt Damon in a cow outfit.) This one is all on Celiac. I thought giving up gluten would be enough, but my entire being tells me differently.

Take care…and be good to my kids!

Fondly,
Gluten Dude

Whole30: When Going Gluten-Free May Not Be Enough

> 2017 Gluten Dude: After doing the Whole30, a light went off in my head that said "this is not just for 30 days, but a lifetime." Not a strict lifetime on the Program, but the mindset that we will NEVER heal unless we take care of our bodies.

I am hitting the restart button on my health…and hopefully on my life. After five years of having celiac disease, things have kinda been sucking lately. I keep waiting and waiting to feel better…to feel normal. And it just ain't happening.

Going gluten-free is simply not enough at this point. My body has been screaming that to me for some time, but I've been too ignorant to listen. The last thing I feel like doing is giving up one food at a time. Too time-consuming and eating is a pain in the ass enough as it is.

So I am giving up everything for the next 30 days. Well…maybe not everything (it just feels that way.)

I got the idea from my good friend Alysa over at InspiredRD. She's been in the same boat as me health-wise and mentioned that she was going on the Whole30 Program in September. I needed something drastic and this was it!

What is the Whole30 Program you say? Basically, for 30 days you eat nothing but "real food" to give your body the chance to heal.

What can I eat? Meat, fish, veggies and fruit.

More importantly, what can't I eat?

Let's start with the two biggies: coffee and alcohol. Let me just say this: I like both of these things very, very much.

(Actually, the program does allow coffee, but since it may possibly be a trigger, I'm giving it up too. As I write this blog, I'm enjoying a hot water with lemon instead of my coffee. And when I say I'm enjoying it, what I really mean is that I hate it.)

What else is forbidden? Grains, dairy, added sugar, legumes and white potatoes. Oh…and of course gluten.

Mrs. Dude and I went food shopping for my journey last night. Holy crap…it's expensive to eat healthy!

Not only am I changing my diet for the next 30 days, but I'm also changing my routine.

Old routine: 5:30 wake-up. Hit snooze repeatedly. Drag my ass to the kitchen to make coffee. An hour on my iPad reading the NY Times, doing the crossword, wasting time. At my desk at 7:30.

New routine: 6:00 wake-up. No snooze. Grab an apple. Head to the gym. Come home, shower and go right to work. Save the iPad until night time.

30 days from now, I am hoping to be revived. Mrs. Dude said recently that I am not the man she married. I'm getting him back!

So today is officially the first day of the rest of my…month.

And to further explain what I can't eat during Whole30, I will explain in "Goodnight Moon" verse. Don't ask me why.

Goodnight Tito's. Goodnight beer.
Goodnight Tequila. Do I make myself clear?

There is no drinking for the entire 30 days.
Will be nice to wake up without my head in a daze.

Goodnight peanut butter. Goodnight rice cake.
My go-to snack I can no longer make.

Goodnight all processed foods. You are not allowed.
Too much of you can put my head in a cloud.

Goodnight sushi. What's that you say??
Rice is a no-no. But sashimi is okay.

What about legumes? Nope, strike 'em off the list.
Nor can I have hummus. I think you get the gist.

After a summer of indulgence, I feel pretty wrecked.
So for 30 straight days, I'll treat my body with respect.

Feel free to join…I'd love the company.
And when the 30 days is up, the first round's on me!!

Change is good. Life is good.

My Whole30 Halftime Report

I have reached the halfway point of my Whole30 Program challenge. After 15 days, here is what I've learned:

I've learned that I needed this. Not just for my health, but for my brain as well. I needed the challenge.

I've learned the results do not come right away. I kept waiting and waiting and was getting beyond frustrated.

I've learned that patience and persistence pays off. As of today (day 18 actually), I'm feeling the best I have in a very long time.

I've learned that eating healthy is not as time consuming as I thought. As long as your fridge is stocked, it takes nothing to cut up some veggies and throw em on the grill or stove.

I've learned that eating this way does indeed cause the weight to drop. I've lost 8 pounds so far.

I've learned to live without sugar in my coffee. I know I said I was going without coffee but I began spending my afternoons working in Starbucks this past week. And when in Rome.

I've learned that by not putting sugar in my coffee, I will be saving a lot of time. You figure it takes an extra 10 seconds to add the sugar and stir it up. Two cups a day is 20 seconds per day. That comes to 7,300 seconds per year. If I live another 40 years, I will have freed up 292,000 seconds. That's 81 days just by not putting sugar in my coffee. What should I do with all my free time??

I've learned that spices are even tastier than sauces and much, much better for you.

I've learned that mornings are much better not hungover.

I've learned that going to the gym at 7:00am gives you the pick of any equipment you want.

I've learned you get a lot more done when you don't nap two hours each day.

I've learned that the mid-afternoon cravings subside being on this program. I'm totally satisfied with my 3 meals and the occasional almond snack.

I've learned that I don't love going to social gatherings without having a cocktail or two.

I've learned Mrs. Dude feels the same way about me (she jokingly refers to the old me as "Fun Bobby"...it's a Friends reference.)

I've learned to LOVE food because it loves me back.

I've learned that eating healthy does not need to be boring.

I've learned that eating healthy does not mean starving yourself.

I've learned that anyone can do this and if you are really struggling with your health, discipline or sanity, this is a great program.

Me Finish Whole30. Eat Like Caveman. Feel Good. You Read.

Gluten Dude finish Whole30.

Gluten Dude really do Whole25.

Gluten Dude lose 12 pounds and me no want lose more. So me stopped.

Me happy with program.

Cave stomach feel better. No ouchie as much.

Gluten Dude learned lessons.

No need rice with meal again, unless Gluten Dude eat sushi.

Rice bad calories that make Gluten Dude tired and full.

No need sugar in coffee. Me now drink black.

No need processed food.

Too many thingies in food not good.

Gluten Dude count ingredients. If more than five, Gluten Dude no eat.

(Gluten Dude only know how to count to five.)

Me like veggies and fruit. Me no miss unhealthy.

Me sleep better when eat like caveman.

Sober caveman not as fun when go to parties in other caves.

Gluten Dude break bad habits.

No need bowl of cereal when sun come up.

Me eat 3 eggs.

No need sugary bar when sun burn bright.

Me eat almonds.

No need to eat til cave stomach full.

Me eat smaller portions.

Overall, Gluten Dude happy.

Cave woman happy too.

Will always eat like caveman now.

Except when outside cave.

Gluten Dude deserve treats once in a while.

Gluten Dude end post now.

Ooops…me forgot to mention (caveman stupid):

Me now eating only cage-free organic eggs and grass-fed organic meat.

Now Gluten Dude done.

Stop Eating Gluten-Free Foods!

2017 Gluten Dude: With over 488 comments (most supportive and some not-so-much), this has been by far my most popular blog post. After the Whole30, I saw the light and wanted to help others. Not everyone shared my views. What about you?

I may not make many friends with the gluten-free food industry with this post, but here goes nothing. And in no way am I telling you what you should do or how you should eat. I just know the pain many celiacs continue to suffer through and I am trying to help the community in any way possible.

I am coming up on my five year anniversary of having celiac disease. In those five years, I can count on one hand the number of stretches where I truly felt healthy. I have suffered stomach pain, severe exhaustion, brain fog, back pain...all of the classic celiac symptoms that I know many in our community continue to deal with.

And in that time, how many times have I eaten gluten? A big fat zero.

So I thought that maybe something else is going on...it can't just be the celiac making me feel this crappy. Multiple doctor visits and test after test came up empty. So then it must be the celiac disease. But if I'm completely gluten-free, why am I still suffering??

Then I heard about the Whole30. It's a program where you eat nothing but whole foods for 30 days; the idea being your body can cleanse itself a bit instead of constantly being in fighting mode as it tries to digest processed foods.

The results for me were nothing less than shocking.

First of all, I lost 12 pounds. My main goal was not to lose weight, as I was only 163 pounds to begin with, but I did want to come down in the 150's. It is absolutely amazing to me that my body shed that much weight simply from eating whole foods.

Second, my energy level is much better than it was. Heck, I don't even nap anymore.

And lastly, my stomach, while not perfect, is much improved.

Based on these results, I am now convinced that celiacs seriously need to rethink the products they are buying and putting in their bodies. We need to get off "eating gluten-free" and replace it with "eating healthy". That will give our bodies the best chance at healing and give us the best opportunity at a normal life.

Here is what my average eating day used to look like:

- Early Morning: Coffee with Splenda and a Kind Bar

- Breakfast: A bowl of Honey Chex with Almond Milk

- Lunch: Brown rice, fish and veggies, cooked with a gluten-free sauce

- Snack: Kind Bar (or some other gluten-free snack)

- Dinner: Gluten-free pasta with chicken, etc.

To me, that looks like a pretty healthy day. But why then did I always feel like crap? Why couldn't I lose any weight at all?

Take a look at the ingredients of Honey Nut Chex when you get the chance. 6 of the first 7 ingredients are pure crap. Is this the stuff celiacs should be putting in their bodies??

Now compare it to an average eating day now:

- Early Morning: Black coffee (no sugar)

- Breakfast: 3 organic eggs with sausage, asparagus, onion and mushroom

- Lunch: Fish and veggies, seasoned with olive oil and spices

- Snack: Almonds or a piece of fruit

- Dinner: A piece of organic chicken or steak with veggies

Two things to take note of:
One...I'm not exactly starving myself.
Two...I'm not eating "gluten-free" anymore.

Let me ask you a question: When you were first diagnosed with celiac disease, what is one of the first things you did? If you're like me, you went to the grocery store and cleaned the shelves of all of the gluten-free items you could find.

"I can't give up pizza!" Phew...I can buy gluten-free pizza.
"I can't give up pasta!" Phew...I can buy gluten-free pasta.
"I can't give up cookies!" Phew...I can buy gluten-free cookies.

You get the point.

The problem is, a large majority of the gluten-free food is absolute garbage. And many (not all) of the gluten-free food manufacturers are more than happy to feed us this crap because they know the emotional attachment people have with eating.

And they know the intense fear celiacs have of losing their lifestyle as they know it. And they know the enormous profit they can make off of us. They don't give a shit about our health.

I've been to a few celiac awareness functions. But you know what? It's not about celiac awareness. It's a damn gluten-free food orgy. It's table after table of foods that celiacs should not be putting in their bodies. But because it's "gluten-free", it must be good for us! Who cares if it's twice as fattening and three times as expensive?

Look…we all deserve treats once in a while and I am not saying you should never eat processed food again. All I'm saying is to give your body a rest…even for 30 days…and see if it makes a difference. And if you are like me, you will never go back to the way you used to eat. There is no reason we should be walking around in pain and simply accepting that's the life of a celiac.

We all deserve to feel good inside.

Got Celiac? Wanna Feel Better? Stop. Eating. Crap.

2017 Gluten Dude: You may be thinking by now: Dang…this guy is really beating a dead horse about eating right. Keep in mind these posts were written over the course of several years. I just packaged them up nicely for your viewing pleasure.

I finished my second Whole30 last week, but before I begin to tell you about how amazing it was (again!), let me get a few things out of the way.

1) I'm not food-shaming anybody here. Just giving some friendly advice as to what worked for me.

2) If you eat poorly and have no desire to change, this post is not for you.

3) If you're struggling with your health but will absolutely not give up [insert treat here] for 30 days, this post is not for you.

4) But if you are low on energy and feeling generally blah, read on and prepare to be transformed (a tad dramatic…I know).

Winter can be a lot of fun, but man is it tough on my body. Thanksgiving leads into our winter vacation, which leads into Christmas, which leads into New Years, which leads into…well…the party continues. By the end of January, my body was begging me to stop. I was tired. Beyond tired. I had trouble focusing at work. I was a beaten man.

And mostly, I got into bad habits (feel free to spank me.) I would have a drink or two a few times during the week. I would grab a gluten-free cookie (or two) here and there. I would have a Hershey bar simply because they were in the fridge. I'd overeat at meals. Individually, none of these things would kill me. But put them all together, and it's a recipe for disaster for this celiac.

At the end of January, Mrs. Dude, who was also feeling the effects of a fun winter, said she was going to do the Whole30. She knows what it did for me the first time I did it. Without even asking me to join her, I jumped at the chance. "I'm in!" And so our 30 day journey began. We toasted ourselves with a gin & tonic and a bag of chips. Just kidding.

The next day, Mrs. Dude took out a second mortgage on our home and went grocery shopping to prepare for our month. We were ready to go.

And now here I am 30+ some days later and I'm telling you, the program is nothing short of amazing. I'm sure you've got questions, so I'll ask them myself.

How hard is it?
That's what she said.

Seriously
You can do anything for 30 days.

Spare us the sound bites. Seriously, how hard is it?
I honestly think it depends on your relationship with food and your desire to change. Since I already gave up gluten and dairy, the switch isn't so tough for me. It's more a mental thing because 30 days does seem like a long time when you are just starting it. "Oh my god…I'm only on day 5??" But eventually, I stopped counting the days.

How did Mrs. Dude do?
I won't speak for her, but she was AWESOME!!!!! It was so much more enjoyable doing it with somebody else this time around. And I was so proud of her.

Didn't you miss eating 'normal' food?
If you are asking me if I missed eating cookies, chips and other treats, the answer is no. It's when those types of foods become part of my daily routine, when they become my normal, I feel like sh*t. Plain and simple.

What did you miss eating?
Sushi. Sashimi is good but just not quite the same for me.

Did you cheat at all?
Food-wise. Not one bit. Beverage-wise? We went to see a friend for a weekend and had a couple of cocktails. No judging please.

How long did it take you to see/feel the results?
By day 3, I felt the best I had in months. I had a clarity about me. I had a lot more energy and focus. I didn't nap for the entire 30 days. I know that sounds ridiculous because what kind of grown man takes naps? But I have a couch in my home office. And on many days, I'd be so tired by the afternoon, that I would literally HAVE TO lie down. For 30 days? Not once!

Did you lose weight?
It wasn't my goal and it shouldn't be your goal, but yes...I lost 6 pounds, mostly the first 12 days.

Now that the program is over, are you back to eating the way you used to?
Not even close.

Isn't moderation the key?
Absolutely. But even some moderation for me affects the way I feel. I'm really trying to be in tune with my body. Those with an autoimmune disease should do the same.

You mean you are never having a cookie again???
Of course I'll have a cookie again. Occasionally. But they will not be a normal staple in our house anymore.

Should I do the Whole30?
I can't answer that for you. Ah hell...sure I can...YES!!

I am always amazed at the power of food and the effect it has on me, both internally and externally. I know what poor eating habits do to my compromised system and I know what it can do to yours too. It's why I cringe when people celebrate the fact that Lucky Charms are now gluten-free. And I cringe even more when some of my fellow celiacs promote it. And it's why I'm disgusted that the Celiac Disease Foundation actually puts their logo on the boxes of Lucky Charms and Cheerios. When our community "leaders" are promoting crap like this, it makes you wonder whose best interest they have in mind.

Look…I know this will fall on a lot of deaf ears. Change is hard. Yes…even when it comes to our health. But I know so many in our community continue to suffer even though we are eating "gluten-free". And I'm telling you, after 30 days of clean eating, it ain't just the gluten that's our issue. It's our food. So stop eating crap if you want to feel good.

AND ONCE AGAIN…WE ALL DESERVE TO FEEL GOOD.

Chapter 4: Eating Out

Eating out. The bane of every celiac's existence. An excursion that used to be something that was looked forward to and fun is now a night of trepidation and anxiety.

Yep…no reason to sugarcoat it…eating out as a celiac can totally suck.

You need to be in a place that you HOPE can keep you safe.

You need to talk to the manager/chef to make sure he or she knows how important it is that your meal be completely gluten-free.

You need to explain to the server about your disease and that you are NOT eating gluten-free because of a fad.

You need to mention cross-contamination and convince them that yes, it CAN get us sick.

You need to scour the menu and find the safest foods.

And even if you do everything right, you may still get sick.

Yeah…kinda takes the joy out of eating out.

But it can be done successfully. I'm living proof of it (even though I have been hit a few times.) You just need to know where to go (find your SAFE spots), what to order and how to handle it.

On the following pages are articles about specific restaurants and what to avoid, personal experiences, wise words from a couple of chefs and overall sound advice on making eating out the best (and safest) experience possible.

Now go make that reservation (even though you'll have reservations.) See what I did there? Ok, now you can proceed.

Dear last night's waiter: I'm gluten free. You're an a**hole.

Dear last night's waiter:

I'm gluten-free...but with all due respect, you're an a**hole. I understand you were busy last night. And I understand it was a Saturday night. And I understand that you want to turn as many tables as possible in the course of an evening (yes...I used to wait tables).

But what was my sin that caused you to cop such a major attitude?

Oh...that's right. I made the grave mistake of telling you that I had celiac disease. And when you didn't know what it was and I told you it was a severe gluten allergy, that was the beginning of the end. Note: I know celiac is not an allergy, but "severe allergy" is easier to understand than "an autoimmune disease where the villi get flattened due to the ingestion of wheat, barley and rye", don't you think?

So you had to make a few extra trips to the kitchen to talk to the chef. So you had to take my "special" order. What's the big deal? Why the eye-rolls? Seriously, you were a total tool.

Believe me...I'm as understanding as they come when it comes to dealing with people with my condition. We celiacs hate having to explain to you what we can and can't have twice as much as you hate having to hear it.

But how about showing a little courtesy? A little heart? A little professionalism? Your job is to take my order, serve my food and make sure I don't get violently ill. And I don't mean that in a degrading kind of way. I have all the empathy and respect for anybody in public service. Dealing with people all day/night can be a real drag. But for now, it's the path you've chosen.

So do me and all of your future customers a favor. Educate yourself a bit. People with celiac disease are not on a diet. We're not trying to lose weight.

We're not part of the new, hip eating fad. And we're certainly not trying to be difficult. Spend a day with me and see what we celiacs go through on a daily basis. It can be pretty tough. So when we go out, we're honestly not looking for special attention. We're not looking to take up too much of your time. Just hear us out and keep us healthy.

And no, that's doesn't mean simply scraping the onion rings off my plate when I remind you I can't have them. But thanks for the big effort just the same.

I like your restaurant. And I'm sure you're a decent guy who was just having a bad night. We've all had them. And if you're my waiter again, I'll give you the complete benefit of the doubt. But if you give me the eye roll again, it ain't gonna be pretty.

Sincerely,

Gluten Dude

P.S. Sorry for the crappy tip. I'll get ya next time.

Gluten & Celiac: A Chef's Perspective

There are always two sides to every story.

And while we as consumers can bitch and moan about gluten, celiac and all the things that come with it, there is an entire industry that is also side-saddled with this problem.

This would be the food industry.

Not the manufacturers of food (who have jumped on the gluten-free bandwagon just fine, thank you) but the chefs who work their butts off each and every day so we can all enjoy a meal out once in a while.

One of my good friends is a personal chef at a vacation home and he has recently opened my eyes to what he goes through on a daily basis as food allergens have become all the rage.

Here is a recent email I received from him:

> "
>
> The issue for people in the food industry is that we deal with people who have this allergy and that allergy and if I eat a speck of dust I will keel over and expire thank you very much. I think they somehow think it makes them more interesting. Then when you are about to serve the offending item to others, all of a sudden it's 'Oh, well, I can have that really – I'll just take a pill" or "Oh, it's my wife (husband) – she thinks I shouldn't have that, but I eat it anyway." This is after you have spent many hours organizing and researching special meals/menus to suit the person with the allergy.
>
> For those with severe allergies and things like celiac disease, this scenario doesn't exist, but unfortunately it is all too common and causes huge irritation and frustration on our part. When we meet

people who have real problems with certain foods it is understandable that we might question it just a teeny tiny bit until we understand the severity of the illness.

I am part of a group on Facebook for chefs. The current huge gripe is people on fad diets – sending their preferences ahead of arrival and specifying what they won't eat. They then proceed to eat and drink anything and everything that is not on the diet. We have had the same thing happen over the years with all the diets you can think of. I once even had a hardcore vegetarian from Michigan who flew all the way here with many wonderful and strange products in her bag that she intended to eat, cluttered up my fridge with them and then never touched. She did remain a vegetarian until the last evening when I was preparing ribs when she then calmly informed me that she would have one. Yes, I was incredulous.

This is what celiacs are up against!

,,

That is what we are up against indeed.

Look…if you read my blog regularly (bless your heart!), you know my mantra is "you are what you eat". I'm a firm believer that diet is the most important thing when it comes to our health, followed very closely by exercise.

And I am all for people giving up certain foods to try to be healthier. And I don't mean the South Beach Diet or any of those other ridiculous money-making fad diets out there. I'm talking giving up real food items to improve your health.

But please…if you are not 100% committed to your food restrictions, think of the person behind the scenes who is working their tail off preparing your food as you requested (note I said "requested", not "demanded"...hint, hint.)

Don't be a pain in the ass if you don't plan on honoring your requests. Respect their time. Respect their skills.

Chefs of the world...unite!

Domino's Goes Gluten Free. Or Do They??

> 2017 Gluten Dude: Domino's was the first major pizza joint to offer gluten-free food. To be blunt…it was a huge sh*t show. And if you are still considering eating there, don't. Nuff said.

How come nothing is ever easy in the celiac world?? Domino's makes an announcement that they are now offering a gluten-free crust and the whole world goes to hell.

I thought my Twitter feed was going to explode yesterday, with opinions coming fast and furious. And boy, did people have strong opinions. There was quite a nice battle going on last night with a few specific parties, who shall remain nameless. I love the passion, but I kept myself out of the loop to give myself some time to mull it over and not react without at least too much emotion.

Here is a quick recap of the situation: Domino's announced yesterday, with a full disclaimer, it will be the first national pizza delivery chain to offer gluten-free crust to its consumers. Domino's partnered with the National Foundation for Celiac Awareness to make sure its gluten-free pizza met the criteria for the foundation's "GREAT Kitchens Amber Designation." This means the ingredients have been verified and managers and staff have been trained on the basics, but kitchen practices may vary with this designation, so *"those with celiac disease and non-celiac gluten sensitivity should ask questions and exercise judgment when dining at an establishment with an Amber Designation."*

In other words, celiacs shouldn't eat it. Flour flying. Cross-contamination. Toppings with gluten. It's a celiac's nightmare.

So the question becomes **"Why did Domino's make a gluten-free crust and promote the hell out of it when it can sicken the people who truly need it?"**

Look…I've always said that celiacs don't own "gluten-free" and companies can do whatever they wish. They are in business to make money. Period. I don't know of one single company that puts their customers over their bottom line. It's always about the profits. Which may explain why the gluten-free option is an extra $3.

So do I think Domino's offered a gluten-free option to truly help those with celiac disease or gluten sensitivity? Of course not. That would make them…human.

(What's that? Corporations are people?? Now I'm really confused.)

And if Domino's gave one hoot about celiacs, they would have made it safe for us. But I've got news for you folks. They don't have to. They make the pizza. We make the choice to eat it or not. And if one celiac eats it, he or she is crazy!

But there are things that trouble me.

For example, why did the NFCA get involved in this if the pizza wasn't going to be safe for celiacs? They actually emailed me directly yesterday and said (in bold no less) that *"Domino's and the NFCA do not recommend it for those with celiac disease."*

Ok…that's cool. They are there to protect us.

But then they finished the email with this: *"We know you are an important blogger and advocate in the celiac community, so we hope you can help us spread the word about Domino's Gluten Free Crust and the steps they're taking to be more transparent."*

Huh? What are they asking me to promote? That Domino's is not really gluten-free?? Again, I just don't quite understand. And then there is this little nugget: On Twitter yesterday, Domino's directly marketed to many celebrities over and over. Here's a sample Tweet:

@GwynethPaltrow Domino's introduced a Gluten Free Crust today. Check here & see if it's right for you.

Puke.

So at the end of the day, Domino's is simply jumping on the gluten-free bandwagon.

Do I hate it? Yes.

Do I think it hurts our cause? Yes.

Have I said this 100 times before? Unfortunately, yes.

Can I blame them? Not really.

But I do have one direct message to Domino's: Be careful what you wish for.

You may have added a full disclaimer, which must have made your legal team do cartwheels in the hallways. But it doesn't mean your message won't get lost in translation. And this could lead to many, many people getting sick.

Note the following tweet from Liz Szabo:

"Domino's to offer gluten-free crust, jumping into $6.2 BILLION marketplace for celiac disease patients."

Note that she said the pizza is for celiac disease patients.

No. No. No, no, no, no no. The pizza is not meant for celiacs. At least not for celiacs who want to survive.

Now, who is Liz Szabo you say? Is she just a misinformed tweeter? A lonely person with an opinion? A mere speck in the Twitter-verse? Nope.

She reports on medical news for USA Today and she has over 15,000 followers. Yep…you read that right. She reports on MEDICAL NEWS for a newspaper that has the widest circulation of any paper in the United States.

And now 15,000 people, 150 of whom have celiac disease, will think Dominos is safe to eat.

And therein lies the problem.

Like I said…it's never easy.

No More PF Chang's for this Celiac

And another one bites the dust.

I have now added **PF Chang's** to the list of restaurants I will no longer eat at. First…a little PF Chang's history. After my celiac diagnosis in 2007, I did not go out to eat for a few months. It was simply too difficult. And then I heard that PF Chang's, which had a location just a few miles from the Dude Ranch at the time, had a gluten-free menu. I love Asian food. I missed eating out. It seemed like a match made in heaven.

I still have vivid memories of that first evening out…

I remember waiting for a table, very anxious about the ordeal. And my little Dudette put her hand on my knee and said "It's ok Daddy. At least you don't have cancer." Little did she know at the time I was just diagnosed with bladder cancer. Mrs. Dude and I had to contain ourselves from breaking out in ironic laughter.

I remember ordering and giving my big celiac speech for the first time. I remember having my first, and last, Red Bridge beer. I remember really enjoying the food, my family and the atmosphere and feeling almost normal.

And I remember thanking the waitress profusely when the meal was over, telling her it was my first time out since my diagnosis and actually tearing up as I was talking to her. To me, it was an emotional experience. She probably thought I was nuts.

The next few times I visited PF Chang's, it was all good. I felt safe (from a gluten point of view), the service was always exceptional, as was the food.

But then little things started happening.

One time, my food came out on the wrong plate. For those who don't understand this, PF Chang's has a different plate for their gluten-free dishes, which I love. But my food did not come out on that plate. So naturally, I questioned my server, who assured me it was gluten-free and was a tad put off that I asked her to go back in the kitchen and verify. It left a poor taste in my mouth.

And then, whenever I'd eat there, I'd start to feel like crap afterwards. I'm not saying I was being glutened (I'm not saying I wasn't either) but I just didn't feel well. I know a lot of their dishes are high in fat and very high in salt, but it shouldn't make me feel this bad. My visits became less and less frequent and Mrs. Dude suggested I stay away from them permanently, which I have.

Until yesterday.

I had a meeting in northern Jersey and was headed back to the Dude Ranch at about 2 in the afternoon. I passed by a PF Chang's and decided to give it a shot. It's amazing how hunger can cloud your judgement. I ordered the gluten-free chicken and broccoli dish with brown rice and told the waitress I was a "severe celiac". I always use the word "severe" when I eat out, hoping it gets them to take me a bit more serious.

My dish came out. Looked good. Took a bite. Tasted fine. But it was really spicy?!? The chicken and broccoli dish is not supposed to be spicy. I asked the waitress about it and she said they put the wrong sauce on it.

You've gotta be kidding me!! She assured me the sauce was indeed gluten-free and came back a few minutes later with the correct meal.

Should I have eaten it at this point? I don't know. But again, I was starving, I was already there and for the most part, I know they take the whole gluten-free thing pretty seriously, so I gave them the benefit of the doubt.

To make a long story short, I ate my lunch and enjoyed the heck out of it.

But as soon as I got in the car, I can't begin to tell you how much my stomach hurt. Beyond painful. And not in a sour stomach kind of way, but in an "alien ready to explode out of my gut" kind of way. The pressure and the tightness were unbearable for the 20 minute drive home.

As soon as I got home, I had to lie down and I ended up sleeping for three hours. I haven't eaten since yesterday's lunch. And this morning, I feel out of it and Mrs. Dude says I look "pasty" (how's that for a visual??).

Now this just shouldn't happen after a lunch out.

So to you PF Chang's…you had me but you lost me. I sincerely appreciate the effort you put in for all celiacs, but our relationship has now come to an end.

I'm not sure what the PF stands for in your name, but for me it now means **Painful Food**.

Sh*t Happens. Don't Let it Ruin the Evening.

I've had celiac disease many years now (yay me!).

In all those years, I have eaten at my brother's house I would say at least 75 times.

My sister-in-law absolutely rocks the house when it comes to cooking for me. When I say she gets it, she seriously GETS IT! It is such a joy to be able to go out and not worry.

But sometimes…stuff happens.

Case in point: Mrs. Dude and I went to their house for dinner Saturday night. The usual amazing gluten-free appetizers for me were put out and we enjoyed a few cocktails. Dinner was going to be steak, potatoes and asparagus. Not just any steak, but "straight from the farm" steak and both rib eye AND filet mignon. Yay me again!

My brother, who was in charge of grilling, was also cooking a non gluten-free marinated pork chop for himself.

I think you can see where this is going.

Dinner is just about ready and my brother walks in from outside with the two steaks and the pork chop…all on the same plate. Oops. And he used the same utensil to cook all of the items. Double oops!!

He simply forgot and truthfully, totally my bad for not reminding him.

My sister-in-law was mortified, my brother felt bad and the night was taking a turn for the worse.

So did I get pissed? Did I throw a tantrum because I couldn't have steak? Did I give him a hard time for cross-contaminating my meal?

Of course I did…I was hungry!!!

Totally kidding. My reaction? Meh…it's only food. And more to the point, it's only ONE meal. Not a biggie.

I've said this time and time again. If you're a celiac, it means rolling with the punches when it comes to food. There are gonna be nights like this one. You have a simple choice to make it better or make it worse.

Always, always, always choose to make it better.

And for the record, the potatoes and asparagus were amazing. As was the after dinner espresso martini and the ping pong.

Life is good.

Are McDonald's French Fries Gluten-Free? Does it Matter?

Dude note: This is not a "Dude on his pedestal" post telling everyone about the evils of McDonald's. We all know they're crap.

Anyway, what this post is about is their French Fries. And not just about whether they are gluten-free or not, but about the risk celiacs are willing to take to eat certain foods.

I follow a specific celiac support group on Facebook. There's some good info. Some bad info. Some fear mongering. Basically what we've come to expect. The other day, someone posted something about eating McDonald's French Fries and feeling awful the next day. My first reaction was "You're a celiac and you're eating at McDonald's??"

But then I realized that some chains supposedly do gluten-free right and maybe I shouldn't be such a judgmental turd.

So I went on the McDonald's website and looked up their fries. And there it is, clear as day: CONTAINS: WHEAT AND MILK. I was actually surprised the first ingredient was potatoes. Who knew they served real food?

Yes, there has been some controversy about these fries within the community. They're supposedly safe in Canada but not in the U.S. But independent testing has shown them to come in below 20ppm in the U.S. But do they use a dedicated fryer? Some locations may and some may not.

My point? It's a huge risk for a celiac to eat their fries.

And what is the reward? [crickets]

So yesterday, I posted on my Facebook page my thoughts on the person eating the fries. It was not a direct attack mind you and of course no names were mentioned. I simply said "A little common sense and education goes a long way toward feeling good. Don't be your own worst enemy."

Good friendly advice right? Well not everyone took it as so friendly.

Some thought I was being way too harsh.

Some thought I was simply wrong and will continue to eat McDonald's French Fries.

Some thought McDonald's was a no go, but Wendy's, Chick Fil A, etc. were ok.

And then there was this stinger: *"Goddamn. I'm glad I'm not a member of this group. What a bunch of judgmental a**holes. This nasty attitude is not only unhelpful, it's harmful. How do you think being mean could be otherwise?"*

Who was being mean? How is telling the truth being an a**hole?

Here's the bottom line folks. You walk into almost any fast food joint, you are taking a gamble with your health. Even if they claim to be gluten-free, there are simply too many risks involved.

And again I ask, what is the reward? [still crickets]

Let's say for argument sake their fries are gluten-free. Great, you say. Well, here are a few quotes from people who have actually worked at McDonald's:

"I worked at mcds for over 6 years up till a couple months ago. They cook them in the same vat as the hash browns. There's wheat in the ingredients anyways. I've had to tell some celiac people coming thru they couldn't have them when they ordered them."

"They cook other things in the fryers when they are busy....I know, my sis use to work at McDonald's."

"My celiac daughter works at our local McDonald's. She sees everything and how it is handled and would not eat the fries or anything on the menu. Ours does not have a dedicated fryer."

So there you have it. Even when it "might" be gluten-free, it seriously "might not" be.

Eating gluten-free is a gigantic pain it the butt. But it ain't rocket science folks.

Please use good judgment and keep yourself healthy.

No reward is worth the risk.

Chipotle Goes Above and Beyond. And Overboard.

We celiacs are a simple bunch. We don't like to cause trouble. We hate being a burden. And man do we miss eating out and not worrying about getting sick. So when we come to your establishment and kindly inform you that we need our meal to be gluten-free, all we ask for in return is honesty and respect.

Honesty...meaning if you cannot provide a safe meal for us, that's totally cool. It's better to know up front. And if you can, kudos to you. Respect...meaning if you decide you can serve us, that you do it quietly and with dignity. We don't like being the center of attention when it comes to our meal.

This brings us to an episode a fellow gluten-free person recently had at a Chipotle in Portland, Oregon. Now, from what I've heard, Chipotle does gluten-free right and their food is good. I personally have never been to one; for the same reason I won't go to almost any chain restaurant. The reward is not worth the risk.

But that's just me. I know many celiacs have had good experiences there. So this is in NO WAY a Chipotle-bashing post. I appreciate the effort they make and also appreciate the warning they put on their website, as follows:

Most people wanting to avoid gluten can eat anything we serve except for our large and small flour tortillas. Everything else is fine to eat for most people wanting to avoid gluten. If you are highly sensitive and would like us to change our gloves, we would be happy to do that at your request. Additionally, because our folks work with wheat tortillas all day long, there may be the possibility of cross-contact in our restaurants. We encourage you to carefully consider your dining choices.

This is perfect. It says "Hey...we get it and we'll try our hardest to accommodate you. But no promises." Like I said, it's all about risk-reward and it's a personal choice.

So taking you back to the whole "honesty and respect" issue, listen to what happened to one of our own recently.

"

Hi Gluten Dude,

First off, thank you for all the advocating you do, especially in light of the surge of recent gluten-free bashing going around. Sadly, I wanted to reach out and share with you an unfortunate and humiliating experience I had today.

Since I am severely gluten intolerant, I am very careful about where I eat out due to medical necessity. One place that I have had good luck at is Chipotle. Their staff is usually well trained and courteous and due to their awareness, I feel fairly safe eating there. Not to mention I really like their values as a company!

I always make sure to very kindly ask them to change their gloves and to have one person take me down the line and apologize for any inconvenience I may cause them and then at the end, I make sure to thank them for their effort. I also try and make every effort to go before peak times so as not to slow the line down and also make it a bit safer for me.

Courteous, right? But even us gluten intolerant folks need to eat.

Well, today I went to the Chipotle located near the Portland, OR airport for lunch and did my usual polite routine only to be met with a confused employee (that's ok!) who went to get the manager, who then made an over the top spectacle of stopping the entire line, and doing more than the usual change of gloves, spoons and quick wipe down.

He had every ingredient batch and every utensil changed, made every staff person on the line step away and wash their hands and change their gloves (instead of just having one person take me the whole way down per usual) and then had them scrub the entire counter length and every single little crevice in between containers. This went on a long time. Then he sent an employee out to the people in line standing behind me who loudly explained that they were sorry for the inconvenience but this person ordering is allergic to gluten so they have to change everything out and offered everyone free drinks as an apology.

If I could have crawled into a crack in the floor I would have. The conversation in the line behind me turned to customers sharing with each other all the negative stereotypes about gluten intolerance.

So while I appreciate Chipotle's usual effort for safety against cross contamination (so important to folks like me and those with Celiac disease), turning it into such a spectacle I was left feeling utterly publicly humiliated and you can bet I will never go into another Chipotle again.

Sad to say goodbye to the tasty food and embarrassed to be gluten-free.

,,

Being the investigative journalist that I am, I asked her the following question: Did the manager do it with a smile? I mean…did you get the sense that he went overboard in order to make a spectacle out of the ordeal, or was he doing it simply to keep you safe?

She said…

" "

The manager smiled and said it was their policy, for my own safety. Which normally I would say yay to! However, I had a hard time gauging his sincerity and his line staff acted quite unhappy to be inconvenienced. I have eaten in many Chipotle locations with a variety of experiences and up until now have always wanted to applaud when they are careful about cross contamination.

This experience felt like a circus act though; exaggerated, prolonged and then sending the staff member out to each of the people in the line behind us to explain I had a "gluten allergy" and offering free drinks to all to make up for up it made me feel like a spectacle.

Neither myself nor my boyfriend noticed anyone in the line grumbling, complaining or acting impatient before then. It was only after that, the line behind us turned pretty hostile with anti gluten-free comments and we couldn't get out of there fast enough.

"

The whole episode seems kind of surreal to me. While there is a part of me that appreciates the effort, something just doesn't sit right about how they handled it. And the bottom line is they made a customer feel so uncomfortable that she'll never eat at a Chipotle again.

So to all restaurants I say this again: We hate this more than you do. YOU think this is a pain in the ass?? Try living with it every single day. If you cannot accommodate us, no hard feelings. If you can, I beg of you to do it with some grace and dignity.

Honesty and respect…not too much to ask for.

How NOT to Treat a Celiac at a Restaurant

What a bizarre and uncomfortable night out I had last Friday. Let me rephrase that. I had a great time with the people I was with, but as far as the celiac stuff is concerned? Total Twilight Zone.

Before the night started, Mrs. Dude and I took a nice walk down to our local wine shop and picked up a nice bottle for dinner. There is a beer store next door. Yes, a beer store. Pennsylvania has these weird, antiquated laws that beer can only be sold in cases from state-owned establishments. Don't ask.

Anyway, we decided to stick our heads in and see if they had any decent gluten-free beer, specifically Glutenberg IPA. They said they had two gluten-free beers. Can you guess which ones? Yep. Omission Beer, which is not even gluten-free beer, and Red Bridge, which sucks.

When I asked if they could get Glutenberg, he laughed at the name of the beer. I walked out embarrassed to be gluten-free. And hence, the night proceeded.

We arrived at the restaurant (since it was 15 miles away, Mrs. Dude and I decided not to walk it) and got seated right away. Now I have been to this restaurant a handful of times. They take their gluten-free seriously and even mark their gfree items on their menu with an asterisk. I've had no issues at any past visit.

Well, I take that back. Last time I was there, I took a picture of the menu and posted it on Facebook (because for some reason, that's what we do nowadays). Many readers correctly pointed out that one of their "gluten-free" items had wheat berries in it. I have no idea how I missed it (and no...I did not order it). I called the restaurant the next day and they were apologetic and said they would fix it right away.

Back to last Friday. When the server first came over, I gave my usual spiel. I told her I have "severe" celiac disease and I will be leaning on her and the kitchen for help. So far…all good.

About three minutes later, another server came over and asked me if I wanted any "celiac bread". Celiac bread? I mean…I knew what she meant, but it just sounded…odd.

I began to peruse the menu. The food at this joint is really, really good. A few of the salads were marked gluten-free. The salad I wanted had fried corn tortillas. I assumed the tortillas were either pre-made or done in a separate fryer. WRONG. They use the same fryer for all of their fried items. The chef said they "try" to do the corn tortillas first. I kindly informed them that the salad should not be labeled gluten-free. No response. For the record, I got another salad and it was amazing.

For the entree, after asking my questions, here is what I ordered: Pan Seared Bronzino Fillet, Roasted Eggplant Puree, White Beans, Chorizo, Artichoke Hearts, Red Pepper Buerre Blanc

The dish came out and I felt myself just staring at it silently. It just seemed to have a lot of "stuff" on it. Mrs. Dude noticed my hesitance and asked the server to come over. I kindly (there's that word again) asked about the sauces on the dish. She said it was fine but if I felt better about things, she could bring the chef out. Very cool.

The chef came out and proceeded to inform me that the dish was fine…there was no flour in it. Now, I would LOVE to assume she knew gluten was more than just flour, but still…

At that point, the waitress said to me "See…you're not going to die." It was said half-sarcastically and half-sincerely, so I had no idea how to process it. I just knew that it made me ungodly uncomfortable.

I know what you're asking now: "Well Dude, did you eat the dish?"

I did. I had been there enough times that, even though the night's experience wasn't a good one, I have not gotten sick there. The meal was spectacular and no, I did not get sick.

At the end of the meal, I thanked my server for looking out for me, as I always do. She then proceeded to tell me that they get so many gluten-free fad dieters nowadays who make a huge deal about their meals being gluten-free but then order the gluten-filled dessert, they just assumed I was one of them until I made it clear I was not.

Can you imagine that? Instead of assuming that I'm eating gluten-free because of a disease, it's the exact opposite. And that's why the gluten-free fad sucks. And that's why restaurants are better off NOT offering gfree unless they are going to do it right. And that's why so many celiacs continue to get sick when eating out.

By the way, I am not going to call out the restaurant publicly. Someone last night was familiar with the menu and said that restaurant used to call their meals celiac safe, but no more. Interesting.

What a night!

The Arrogance and Ignorance of Panera Bread

Tom Gumpel is the head baker for Panera Bread. Panera Bread has decided to jump into the gluten-free TREND. Tom Gumpel is not happy about this. This does not bode well for the celiac community.

Arrogance and ignorance are not our friend (are they anybody's friend??)

Let's start with the arrogance.

Here are some of Mr. Gumpel's quotes:

"Bread has been just beaten up. You have 10,000 years of bread in some form or function, and then all of a sudden this generation has just killed it. Whether it's the carbohydrates, low-carb, gluten [free], pick something." (entrepreneur.com)

That's right Tom…this health-conscious generation is just killing the bread industry. Silly us trying different things so we can feel better. Adapt or find another job.

"There are some pretty poor gluten-free breads out there, so I went into this kicking and screaming. Once I committed to it, I said to myself, 'how would you pull this off as an artisan baker?' There is little to no good-tasting gluten-free bread in this country, and I've eaten about every slice there is. We are responding to peoples requests and doing it with integrity." (thedailymeal.com)

Thanks so much Tom for coming to our rescue. We've been waiting for someone just like you to FINALLY deliver real gluten-free bread. You're my hero!!!

Wait…hold on…my inner voice is saying something. What's that? There are other companies out there already making good gluten-free bread? Like gfJules, Jennifer's Way, Three Bakers, Canyon Bakehouse?

Ah…never mind Tom, you're not my hero. You actually sound like a misinformed egomaniac. Please…don't do me any favors.

Moving onto ignorance.

Panera is making the gluten-free bread with 100% gluten-free ingredients. Yay…it's gluten-free!

Panera is making the gluten-free bread in a gluten-free facility. Yay…it's gluten-free!

Panera is displaying and storing the gluten-free bread next to the regular menu items. What??

They are not even calling it gluten-free. They are calling it…ugh…gluten conscious.

Gluten conscious. Let that sink in a bit.

So let me get this straight…you don't WANT to do this, you feel like you HAVE to do this; you are taking all of the right precautions in baking the bread, but then cross-contaminating the hell out of it; and then you're coming up with a ridiculous term for it, making it that much more difficult for the celiac community to be taken seriously.

Look…I've said hundreds of times that celiacs don't own gluten-free. Panera Bread is a business. And the number one goal of any business is to make money. And they will do whatever it takes to reach that goal. But please don't act like you are doing the world a big favor and lowering your standards so you can appease the gluten-free community.

Speaking for myself…I'm just not that desperate for your bread.

Consider this a "conscious uncoupling".

What to do if You've Been Glutened Eating Out

Now as most of you celiacs know, going to a restaurant can be an adventure in fear and anxiety. Really takes about half the fun out of eating out. Now let's assume you get glutened from a restaurant. What do you do? What are your next steps? How do you respond?

Here's an interesting email I recently received that asks these same questions. See below for my thoughts.

> "
>
> Dude — thanks for all the advice over the last 2/12 years since I was diagnosed w celiac. Have not seen this topic addressed on your sites: what do you do when you get glutened at a restaurant? This occurred at a rock-solid reliable favorite — it was crazy busy, not the best of circumstances and stuff happens.
>
> Do you contact the restaurant as a teachable moment? Do you let it go? File a complaint? Your experience and insight are appreciated.
>
> "

Short answer: Yes. Kind of. No.

Long answer: While lord knows I've been hit over the years from eating out, there is only ONE time where I knew a restaurant effed up. Because they told me...as soon as I took my last bite. What proceeded was six months of hell. Yes...six months.

And what did I do with regards to the restaurant? A big, fat nothing.

What should I have done? Good question. Though looking back, I cannot believe I paid for my meal.

So here's my advice. Unless you are 100% sure the restaurant glutened you, I don't think you say anything. You don't want to be accusatory unless you have facts to back you up. If you are indeed positive they messed up, yes, you definitely ask to speak to the manager or owner and let them know. It's a teachable moment indeed and if you can prevent the next celiac from getting sick, at least some good may come out of it.

And then yeah…you let it go. No need to carry it around with you. Getting glutened is exhausting enough. Carrying the anger along with it won't help you heal.

Do you file a complaint? This gets a big "it depends" answer. In your situation…no. Like you said, their game is usually on. But if the restaurant is callous about gluten-free, if they are not taking any precautions regarding cross-contamination, if their reason for offering gluten-free seems to be profit over people, then heck yeah, file away.

My two cents. Agree? Disagree? Do tell.

I Will **NOT** Say Thank You (a letter to a waitress who mocked my disease)

Dude note: Sometimes emails sent to me need no introduction. Just read and absorb.

"

To the waitress(es) who mocked me for ordering gluten-free:

This is not a thank you letter.

You know the kind. The social media posts that call out a social injustice, but in turn end up "thanking" the culprit for some sort of inspirational reason. Honestly, I thought about wording this in that way. Then I thought about the way it felt when you openly mocked my disease.

The same way it feels when I see people do it in the media. The same way it feels when I read about children getting bullied at school for the same reason.

I will not say thank you.

We only met once, as your shift was over shortly after you took our order. You don't know much about me, or I about you.

What you don't know is that I could hear you. You were right behind me — or was that the point?

What you don't know is that the words you and the other(s) were saying are the exact words I fear the staff is thinking every time I go out. Are they taking me seriously? Will the food be safe? Will I spend the next 12-24 hours violently ill and have my intestines damaged because I took this risk of going out?

What you don't know is that I didn't want to ask you all those questions. I long for the days I could look at a menu and order simply and without fear.

What you don't know is that what one of you labeled as "attention-seeking behavior," is actually considered "unwanted visibility" in the Celiac community. Having to explain my disease can be and is emotionally exhaustive.

I will not say thank you.

What you don't know is that there are millions of people with Celiac Disease. MILLIONS.

What you don't know is what it's like to feel like a burden to your friends and family because of something you can't control.

What you don't know is what it's like to be afraid of food.

What you don't know is what it's like to constantly wash your hands every day, praying you don't get sick when you touch your food.

What you don't know is what it's like to never relax.

What you don't know is that my mind can never shut down from thinking about gluten-free. You see, my life literally depends on it.

What you don't know is that I will never again in my entire life be able to eat something without doing FBI-like research on it to know if it's safe.

I will not say thank you.

What you don't know is what it's like to go to any social event and know that you can't eat a single thing there.

What you don't know is the overwhelming feelings of both gratitude and isolation when a friend or family member goes out of their way to bring food to that social event that is safe for you to eat.

What you don't know is that my husband had to very thoroughly brush his teeth after our meal before he could kiss me again, because a simple kiss on lips that have touched gluten is dangerous for my body.

I will not say thank you.

What you don't know is that I have to endure jokes about gluten-free every single day.

What you don't know is the feeling of those jokes going straight to my (albeit sensitive) heart, knowing that the most serious, dangerous part of my life, the thing that I cannot afford to stop thinking about, is a punchline.

What you don't know is that I wish I could have said these things to your face. Not to be aggressive or mean, but to simply get the words out. Simply to let one more person know that Celiac Disease is real and it's not easy.

What you don't know is that I'm not angry with you; you simply just don't understand.

You may have actually known some of these things. I wouldn't know that, though, because we only met briefly.

I don't know anything about your life. I'm sure you have struggles; everyone does. This is mine.

So no, I will not say thank you. There is not some grand inspirational lesson learned in this. This is my every day life, and it will only get worse unless people tell the world what it's like to live with Celiac.

And that's what I plan to do.

"

Papa John's and Starbucks Go Gluten-Free. Let's Take a Look.

It ain't easy being a celiac. And for restaurants, it ain't easy to feed us. I get that.

And I also get that any time we eat out, unless the restaurant is 100% gluten-free, we take a risk. It's a risk I'm willing to take, though I err way, way, way on the safe side. For example, you'll never see me at a fast food joint. One because the food would rot my gut to pieces; two because most of it tastes like crap; and three because there is no way in hell I'm putting my faith in that kind of environment (cross-contamination galore, kids working, etc.)

But I know everyone is not like me.

Dude note: When I was a young lad (with no friends mind you and bullied on a pretty regular basis), I always thought: "Why can't everyone be just like me? The world would be so much better." You might call it confidence. I call it ignorance. Anyway, back to business.

And I know for lots of reasons (convenience, money, etc.) our community will continue to eat at these joints. No judgment here. Promise. And when the joints do it right, I give them credit and when they do it wrong, I give them hell. Right Dominos and Panera??

All I know is that when a restaurant offers gluten-free, they have a responsibility to DO IT RIGHT. I always say celiacs don't own gluten-free and I have no problem with ANYBODY going gluten-free. They have their reasons. But as my partner in crime Jennifer Esposito once said:

"People need to understand this is a serious disease. And when you ask for gluten-free in a restaurant and you are not gluten-free; the more we have people not being able to decipher if this is an allergy, a fad or a disease, our community is getting sicker and sicker and sicker. I ask you to be responsible about this disease. I am asking that people

be responsible and respectful for the people that suffer with this disease. It is not fun. It is not easy. And it is not a fad."

God…I love that.

Right now you're probably wondering if I'm ever gonna get to the point. I feel your pain. Here we go.

Two chains recently announced they are offering gluten-free items: Papa John's and Starbucks. I'll take them one at a time. This time there will be judgment. Promise.

Starbucks Goes Gluten-Free!?

This is actually big. I like Starbucks. I don't love their coffee, but I like their vibe, their fight for causes I believe in and the fact they pay their people fairly. But their big drawback is, not only have they never offered gluten-free food on their menu, there is absolutely no way to know if there is gluten in any of their drinks (except black coffee). It's not listed anywhere in the establishment and it's not on their website. For a company that large, it's actually surprising it took them this long to jump in.

So did they do it right? It's time for a little Q & A with myself.

Dude note: See…when you have no friends, you tend to have conversations with yourself. Some habits are hard to break.

Don't you and Mrs. Dude play "The Starbucks Game", when you can see who can spot the most Starbucks when you're in NYC?
How did you know?

Lucky guess. Ok…what is Starbucks offering?
A Gluten-Free Smoked Canadian Bacon & Egg sandwich

What are the ingredients?
The less you know…the better. Let's just say there are A LOT of them. But no gluten.

How do they keep it safe from cross-contamination?

From their website: *It's all prepared in a certified gluten-free environment and sealed for your safety. We then warm and serve it in its own oven-safe parchment bag to avoid any cross-contamination.*

So it's totally safe for celiacs?

This is where it gets a bit tricky. Even though they say it's made in a certified gluten-free environment, on the very same web page it says this: *"We cannot guarantee that any of our products are free from allergens (including dairy, eggs, soy, tree nuts, wheat and others) as we use shared equipment to store, prepare and serve them."*

Yeah…I know. Maybe just a CYA statement, but not really sure.

So do you think it's safe?

Man, you ask a lot of questions.

Sorry, I'm a curious man-child.

That's ok. Me too. I've read other celiacs' reviews and it mostly seems like they are doing it right. A few times, the counter person erroneously removed the bag or they unsealed the bag before heating it up. But that just comes from proper training and being a smart celiac by keeping an eye on things behind the counter. As for the taste, again from what I've read, it's nothing special but it's not awful. Others can chime in here.

Last question. Will you try it?

Probably not. Not necessarily because I think it's unsafe, but 1) it's got cheese (me no eat dairy) and 2) based on the ingredients, I just have a feeling it would sit in my stomach like a rock. But I'm not condemning Starbucks. They sure as hell did it better than Papa John's.

Papa John's Goes Gluten-Free!?

I'm not gonna spend too much time on this one.

It's a personal size pizza and they say the crust is prepared in a gluten-free environment before going to the stores. But this is directly from their site:

165

Papa John's does not recommend pizzas with Papa John's Ancient Grains Gluten-Free Crust for customers with Celiac Disease. Although Papa John's Ancient Grains Gluten-Free Crust is gluten-free and Papa John's employs procedures to prevent contact with gluten, it is possible that a pizza with Papa John's Ancient Grains Gluten-Free Crust is exposed to gluten during the ordinary preparation process. Please use your best judgment in ordering a pizza with Papa John's Ancient Grains Gluten-Free Crust if you have a sensitivity to gluten.

They can absolutely make it as they wish. They are in business for profit. And making really awful commercials with Peyton Manning. But what I don't understand is if it's not made for people who have sensitivities to gluten, THEN WHO IS IT MADE FOR?

And I know what's gonna happen. Too many celiacs will see gluten-free at Papa John's and order a pizza without thinking twice. They'll get sick and Papa John's will be none the wiser. And that just sucks.

Like I said, it ain't easy being a celiac.

Chapter 5: It's All About the Attitude

"If you don't like something, change it. If you can't change it, change your attitude."
– Maya Angelou

"The greatest discovery of all time is that a person can change his future merely by changing his attitude."
– Oprah Winfrey

"It is very important to generate a good attitude, a good heart, as much as possible. From this, happiness in both the short term and the long term for both yourself and others will come."
– Dalai Lama

"You've got to learn to live with what you can't rise above."
– Bruce Springsteen

Have I made my point yet? Attitude is EVERYTHING when it comes to dealing with celiac disease. With a bad attitude, you're a dead man walking. A good attitude will lead to a happier and healthier life.

You got celiac? You struggling? Read the following, learn from me and from the community, rise above it and you'll be looking at the bright side in no time.

No…really you will!

Dear Celiac Newbies: Patience, Patience, Patience (and don't eat crap)

Do you know one of the main reasons I started this blog four years into my celiac journey?

Because almost everyone said it would be easy. And it's not.

Because almost everyone said I'd feel better right away eating gluten-free. And I didn't.

Because celiac is such a puzzle to solve. And I didn't have all of the pieces. And fact is...I still don't. But I'm in such a better place than I was four years ago.

It's rare that I write a blog post two days in a row (I'm very aware of Dude Fatique). And it's rarer when I receive an email from a newly diagnosed celiac that is in such anguish, that I'm drawn to respond right away. But the email I just received calls for such an occasion (damn...I misspell "occasion" every single time. Thank you auto-correct!).

Here's the email I just got...

> "
>
> From Starving in NY
>
> I was diagnosed with Celiac Disease about a week and a half ago and it has been a long journey to stay the least. I am now 36 and my problems started when I was 19 years old. I have had numerous blood tests, colonoscopy and an endoscopy coming up soon. I have been told, throughout the years, that my blood work is negative and at other times borderline for Celiac Disease. Well...the last results were positive. I'm a mess and I'm actually crying while typing this email as I sit in my cubicle at work.

I'm beyond tired of feeling like my insides are constantly rebelling against me. I cannot take it anymore…no one should have to live like this. I have tried a gluten-free diet in the past, but I still have had terrible sickness. I know now that I have no choice but to stay on a gluten-free diet for the rest of my life, so the day I got the call that I had a positive result, I started it up again.

At first I felt a significant amount of relief, but for the last 3 days I have felt terrible. I feel like when I eat gluten I am a sick, but I also am sick on a gluten-free diet. I'm totally at the end of my rope and tempted to give up on food completely. I just don't understand what I'm doing wrong.

I know that there are people out there that have it much worse, but I guess I'm just feeling like I'm at a crossroads with food. Damned if I do…damned if I don't. I'm really not looking for a reply…I just needed to vent this out. Besides, I think this email is bit of a crazy rant and I apologize for any grammatical errors…not in a good way at the moment.

Thanks for listening.

"

There is no need to starve…I assure you. First things first, do not go gluten-free until AFTER your endoscopy. Otherwise, it may not be accurate. So try to get that done asap.

My first big piece of advice: Be patient. It can take the body months/years to heal completely. It's not going to happen overnight. I know that sucks because you've been feeling awful for so long. Stay the course.

Here is the one thing I wish people told me upon my diagnosis: Going gluten-free is just one part of the puzzle. Yes, it hopefully allows your body to begin to heal. Yes, it is the ONLY treatment for our disease. And yes, it is indeed step one in your recovery. But did you know that four years into my gluten-free diet, I still felt like crap. Or as Mrs. Dude always accurately said…"YOU NEVER FEEL WELL!" As always, she was right.

So the question is…why didn't I feel well? I was doing what the doctors said. I was doing what many in the community said. And yet, I felt just as bad as the day I was diagnosed (even though my body was indeed healing…as I put on the 15 pounds that I lost the year before my diagnosis).

So what did I do to begin my new journey? I stopped eating gluten-free. Meaning I stopped buying replacement foods and started eating food food. Yes, I said food twice. There is such a fear for the newly diagnosed of giving up all of the things they once loved. Don't get me wrong. Eating crap once in a while is fun; but not while your body is still damaged from

It's not easy to hear, but I believe it's important.

There is no "one size fits all" for celiac disease. Your disease is not my disease. It all affects us differently and we all must find out what works for us.

Celiac disease is a true puzzle and it can take years to get all of the pieces to fit together. Be patient. And then be more patient. And in the meantime, don't be too hard on yourself and by all means don't give up. You'll get there.

Change "I Can't Have That" to "I Don't Want That"

"I can't have that??" has now been replaced in my vocabulary with "I don't want that" and man does it feel good.

I heard these phrases written by one of my fellow tweeters and it really resonated with me. It is a complete eating mentality shift that has taken place that has brought so much peace (and health) to my life and if you can make the adjustment, it will to yours too.

When I was diagnosed with celiac disease, and for several years afterwards, my entire focus was always on what I couldn't eat. I was in mourning for the loss of so many foods that I enjoyed.

"No beer?"

"No pasta?"

"Seriously, no beer??"

And, hey, it's ok to mourn. For a bit. But after a certain point, it is completely self-defeating.

Not only are the foods you must give up making you sick, but many of them were most likely not too healthy in the first place. Why would you want to go back to that previous life?

I am currently in the best shape of my life. Yes, I exercise. Yes, I was blessed with skinny genes. But if I didn't have celiac disease and I was still eating the foods I used to eat, I'm sure the story would be quite different.

So stop dwelling on what you can't have.

Stop feeling sorry for yourself.

You've been given the gift of celiac disease.

What you do with that gift is up to you.

Repeat After Me: It's Only Food

Yeah…having celiac disease can be a total drag. I'm in the midst of two weeks of hell from who knows what. So in no way am I minimizing how difficult our disease can be to live with. I detest this disease with every fiber of my being.

But I'll be honest with you. I have very little tolerance for people who intentionally cheat (eat gluten) and then have the stones to complain about how bad they feel.

I see it on Twitter all the time. Crap like *"Should have known better but that bagel looked so good. #celiacsucks"*. Please. That brings us to a new celiac rule (haven't had one of these in a while): If you intentionally eat gluten, there is absolutely no complaining about it. Period.

This leads me to a comment that was recently left on my blog post about lymphoma and celiac disease. At first, I was going to ask for the community's support for this fellow celiac who is having a hard time staying gluten-free. You know… *"rah, rah…you can do it…we're all behind you."*

But when I read the comment again this morning, it just hit me differently. Yeah, I know food can be addictive. Yeah, I know having to give up gluten for LIFE is a bummer. But at the end of the day, IT'S ONLY FOOD. Not only that, but it's only SOME food. There is still SO MUCH we can eat. I always tell people, the food is probably the easiest part about having celiac disease. It's all the other crap that goes along with it that makes it such a pain in the ass to live with.

So you can't have a NY bagel. So you can't have a nice 90 minute IPA. So you can't have a slice of pizza on the run.

A bummer? You bet.

A tragedy? Not even close.

Am I being too harsh on this woman? Here's her comment. You tell me.

"

You know the actor who died recently from a heroine overdose – I cannot remember his name. Sometimes I identify with what it might have been like for him. "I know this might kill me, but I just can't stop."

I googled, "celiac and cheating" to get a refresher in how this effects my body. I am scared. I am very aware and still I feel like I cannot stop especially during PMS.

I have two beautiful children with many food sensitivities. My whole life is food. I know I need to be a good example. Many of you are likely aware of how gluten and dairy effect the opiate receptors. I feel like I need an addictions specialist. I am sharing this because I hear the judgment and disbelief that someone would do this to themselves. It is horrible and I am ashamed.

I think for some of us it may be more complicated. It does not feel like simply making a choice. Some days I feel like every moment I am fighting a craving. If my attention and will are pulled in a different direction (which is often with a toddler and a husband who travels for work), I become weak. I know there are answers and I am committed to figuring it out. I am sharing just in case anyone else has felt like this….you are not alone.

I also express much admiration for those who just decide they are done – and that's it. I cannot eat dairy, any grains, nuts, seeds, eggs, soy, or night shades. It is not an excuse. I must figure it out. It is difficult. My cheating has nothing to do with a lack of love for my family but some crazy out of control compulsion in my head.

I am not asking anyone to understand….just letting you know what it might be like for some of us. Very much like the alcoholic who drinks and knows if he doesn't stop, he might lose everything.

"

I feel for this woman. She is obviously struggling. I'm glad she felt comfortable enough to share her message with us and I truly wish I had an answer.

But I'm just not in an "It's ok…I understand how tough it is" mood.

Perhaps she needs to hear from people who have a gentler message.

This morning…that just ain't me.

With Celiac Disease, Attitude is EVERYTHING

I follow a few celiac ~~complaint~~ support groups on Facebook. I don't comment at all…I just like to see what kind of issues my fellow celiacs are dealing with. Lots of great people with legit concerns but I swear, sometimes it's like being at a "whiners" convention. Or better yet, an "I shouldn't have taken the risk and eaten that, but I did and now I feel awful" convention.

Every so often, I'm tempted to pipe in and lend some celiac advice, but I remain an outsider instead (story of my life). But everyone who has celiac disease should read an email I received last week from a 12-year-old celiac whose spirit and attitude lifted my spirits and I thought she provided a great example of how we should all look at celiac disease.

The letter is beautifully written and another lesson to all of us adult celiacs how to tackle not only our disease, but life itself. Sometimes it sucks, but it is what it is.

❝

Dear Gluten Dude,

I am 12 years old. I was diagnosed with Celiac in the second grade. I'm now in sixth grade. I have only gotten sick from gluten 5 times in the last 5-6 years. I sometimes wish that I wasn't gluten-free or really actually all the time. Because at parties and gatherings I have to bring all my food. And sometimes I get made fun of…a lot.

I know that people don't understand Gluten but I mean I don't understand why some people would try to put other people down because of something that they can't control. In third grade this girl dared me to eat a roll at school (which wasn't gluten-free) i said no, then she asked why. So I told her it would make me sick. Then she literally tried to put that roll in my mouth.

In 5th grade I was at this place and we were all going to the pool and I asked this girl if I could swim with her and she was like no. The water isn't gluten-free. And she laughed in my face.

I think some people don't know how hard it is. I mean I know it isn't cancer but it sure is hard. I haven't had this certain looking macaroni in like 3 years. But I'm okay with that.

So to all those little kids and adults out there who are sad or upset because other kids make fun of you or just because the fact of Gluten Free is sad already to you, just remember that God gave you this because he has a purpose for you. I hope all Gluten Free people have every meal as your best just because it's special for you.

"

Just. Love. It.

I'm Going to a Gluten-Filled Party....and I Can't Wait

If I've said it once, I've said it more than once, **celiac is all about attitude**. If you let celiac dictate your life, you're screwed. If you let food become more important than people, you're toast (pun sort of intended). If you carry the celiac burden with you at all times, you are simply missing out on life.

Case in point...my awesome sister-in-law is having a milestone birthday next week. So my just-as-awesome brother is throwing her a big bash this Saturday at their house (you're all invited by the way). All my brothers coming in, her family making the trip, my Aunt coming down from CT.

And there will be food. Lots and lots of food. He is having the party catered. None of the food will be safe for me to eat...and I couldn't be happier about it.

Happy...because my sister-in-law, who always goes out of her way to keep me safe, can remove that from her plate for one night.

Happy...because it's less worrying for me (will it REALLY be ok for me to eat??)

Happy...because it's less work for the caterers (how do I keep things separate? Did I use the right utensil??)

Happy...because Mrs. Dude can relax and not worry about me getting sick.

Happy...because I didn't have to put my brother out in any way.

I know what you're saying. Sure Dude, you're happy but won't you...um...you know...be HUNGRY??

Nope. Because along with "attitude", the second key word in celiac success is "preparation".

Mrs. Dude and I put together an awesome meal plan. Ok...let me rephrase that. Mrs. Dude put together an awesome meal plan.

When everyone else is having appetizers, I'm having a small gluten-free pizza.

When everyone else is having soup and salad, I'm having sushi.

When everyone else is having their main dish, I'm having fish and veggies.

When everyone else is having dessert, I'm having a homemade gluten free brownie.

My point is...I'm not exactly going without, am I? I'm prepared as prepared can be and have a can't wait attitude. If I can do it, so can you.

Happy Birthday Beth-Anne. Let the party begin!

To All Celiac Newbies: Don't Beat Yourself Up

We were all newly diagnosed at one time or another. And we all messed up. Every single one of us.

It's a brand new world when you're diagnosed and there is simply no way in hell you make the transition unscathed.

Heck…it's years later and I can still eff up sometimes.

My advice to newbies…give yourselves a break. We're only human.

Here's an email I received from a newbie who is beating herself up pretty good.

> "
>
> I am newly diagnosed with Celiac disease (3 months in) and thought I was at least at the point where I wasn't crying in frustration over it anymore, but here I am struggling to see the keyboard because I am crying again. Over chili. Over gluten-free organic chili in a can that made me sick today. Chili labelled gluten-free but processed in a facility that also processes wheat. And I missed that on the label. I am so going to pay for this with exhaustion and achy joints for weeks.
>
> I can't take off work to rest. I used up too many sick days getting the diagnosis and then finding a GI who had a clue about this damned disease. I need the rest of my days for the next round of appointments to deal with all the other weird symptoms cropping up. Not to mention I feel absolutely ridiculous saying that I need to stay home because I ate the wrong chili!
>
> I know I am lucky. Lucky I didn't die from the perforated intestine that led to this diagnosis. Lucky I have supportive friends and family.

Lucky that (so far) my limited forays into local restaurants have been positive with no rolled eyes and no getting sick for me.

But today I am crying over chili and my own stupidity. Because as much as I have read about this disease and how careful to be, I know I have injured myself when I am trying to heal. And I hate that I did that. Just as I hate this disease.

I get worn out sometimes trying to keep myself safe and healthy. I don't miss any particular food from before diagnosis and nothing could make me cheat, but oh how I miss convenience and ease! They are missing from my life these days and when even gluten-free organic chili is out to get you....well, today I cried. Again.

"

As I said above, we've all been there so you're in good company. It's an adjustment period, no doubt.

Give yourself a break. I know it's crappy getting sick. The physical aspect of it is bad enough. Don't emotionally pile on yourself. It will just make it that much worse.

And just remember...there's no crying.

Chin up.

75 Reasons to Love (??) Celiac Disease

You better believe I put the question marks after the word "love" in my title. Do I love my disease? Heck no. I pretty much detest it. It's a constant unwanted companion in my life.

That being said, it's time to shed some positive light on our disease. Without further ado, here are 75 reasons to love (there's that word again!!) celiac disease. Oh…and tons of thanks to the celiac community for their input. Many of the reasons below came from my fellow celiacs. (What…you thought I could come up with 75 on my own???)

1. I got my life back now that I no longer feel like crap all the time.

2. I don't have to go out for lunch with clients I don't like anymore!

3. It's a disease treatable by food. No reliance on the pharmaceutical industry.

4. It's made me much more aware of what I put into my body (and what I don't!)

5. I found out who my true friends are (those who believe & respect my needs), as well as those who just think I'm full of crap.

6. I GOT MY LIFE BACK!!!

7. The great community of people like yourself, Jules Shepard, Jennifer Esposito etc. who are in the trenches and doing so much to educate us.

8. Celiac has made me much more aware that people are struggling with things that I may never know about or understand.

9. I am finally healthy enough to exercise.

10. Learning that there is more to life than food.

11. I have learned to LISTEN to my body.

12. I now have the ability (forced education though it was) to successfully cook more than a baked potato.

13. I promote my boyfriend's dental health since he has to brush his teeth before kissing me.

14. I love knowing what caused me so much anguish throughout my childhood and young adulthood.

15. If you are what you eat, I'm difficult, I'm complicated and I'm really, really expensive! But so much better!

16. Now that I know what foods make me sick, I feel free to be more adventurous and try new things that I know are gluten-free.

17. I love that I'm not sick every day.

18. BACON!!!

19. Being a survivor of Celiac disease, rather than a victim of it, translates into other areas of my life.

20. My cooking repertoire has increased exponentially!

21. I don't have to eat the endless office treats and don't get guilted into eating them.

22. I always have the perfect excuse to refuse all those horrible foods that everyone makes for pot lucks.

23. I get to have so many people ogle over the fact that I have such great "self-control".

24. Celiac disease makes you a great judge of character. You want to rant about my "fad diet" choices while I watch you eat bread? Something tells me we won't be the best of friends.

25. You alone control what you eat, what you eliminate, how much you learn and how pro-active you become.

26. Vodka…gluten-free. Tequila…gluten-free. Gin…well, you get the point.

27. Simply three numbers, 129. That's how much I weighed in yesterday at the Dr's office. This time last year I was 98lbs.

28. I really thought it was cancer…all my horrible symptoms. Turns out it's the food I'm eating. Yay!!!! It's celiac disease!

29. We have Gluten Dude! (I had to throw this one in the article.)

30. I have a valid excuse for not eating my mother in law's horrible cooking.

31. Nothing beats the relief of actually knowing that there was truly something going on with my body.

32. It means saying goodbye to 35 years of migraines.

33. You think outside the BOX….which means, you do not eat from a BOX….real food.

34. After three miscarriages, I was diagnosed with cd and we now have a beautiful 2 year old daughter.

35. Celiac has forced me into to becoming a dynamite home chef!

36. I can still have chocolate and wine.

37. Two words: ICE CREAM.

38. There are millions of people who feel tired, depressed, and exhausted and yet they do not know why. We know.

39. Having a better education on how food really affects my body.

40. Celiac disease took my mom's life. Getting a diagnosis saved mine.

41. Celiac disease introduces you to a new community of friends.

42. It puts you in a position to be able to help and encourage others to get tested.

43. The relief of having a diagnosis and not being told it is all from stress.

44. If it weren't for celiac disease I'd still be eating garbage under the illusion that it doesn't affect my body.

45. Celiac disease weeds out the idiots in your life.

46. It has taught me and now my daughters, to roll with the punches, get up, dust yourself off and get creative.

47. Without gluten, there aren't horrifying mood swings and depression that makes you feel like you are going to crawl in to the earth and become part of the mud.

48. Not having to politely take one of the sketchy looking cookies your coworkers bring in.

49. Our celiac children will learn to put a positive spin on all situations rather than be taught to complain and be negative.

50. It's no longer "I shouldn't". It's now "I can't".

51. It empowers me to raise my voice and speak out for myself.

52. Cooking at home also leads to sitting down around a table and eating together as a family.

53. Knowing "it's not in my head!!"

54. It forces me to read labels even more closely.

55. Eating right has given me the energy to enjoy an active life!

56. My organism only accepts good food, organic, grass fed, fresh ingredients…Is this really a disease or a blessing?

57. Sushi. Sushi. Sushi. You just need to know what to order.

58. I have met people and visited places that I would never have seen otherwise!

59. It helps me understand people with other health challenges better and have more patience and empathy.

60. I actually enjoy eating now because it doesn't hurt like hell anymore.

61. It took the "option" of self-control off the table.

62. There are FINALLY some great gluten-free beers on the market. Cheers to that!

63. Hello, celiac and gluten-free diet. Goodbye, asthma and freak show skin problems.

64. I fell in love with food – real, whole, living food – after going gluten-free and would not trade it for the world.

65. It made me much more aware of sneaky ingredients in food—not just gluten containing ones.

66. I can avoid foods that I don't like that are pushed on me. Damn…those [insert food you hate here] are breaded!? Bummer

67. Walking by the bakery section of a grocery store and having absolutely no desire for anything there.

68. After lots of trial and error and epic failures in the kitchen, when you finally produce a delicious baked good, it feels like you've conquered the world!

69. When you go to a social gathering, you don't have to try Aunt Sally's newest lime Jell-O, pretzel, celery combo....with Cool Whip.

70. I now have a legit reason not to attend outings/get togethers with people I didn't like in the first place.

71. It can be an incredible screening tool for relationships.

72. It teaches patience since the healing process is slow and requires commitment.

73. I now have no problem telling people NO and fully advocating for myself which has spread to many aspects of my life.

74. It proved that I'm not a hypochondriac.

75. It beats dying!

So there you have it folks. Yeah...celiac disease sucks. No...of course most of us don't "love" it. But don't let it drag you down. Embrace it, accept it and go on living your life.

And on those days you are struggling, just remember...WE CAN HAVE SUSHI AND TEQUILA!

Chapter 6: Relationships (or lack thereof)

I'm not going to lie to you. I'm blessed. I'm more than blessed. The people I surround myself with are friggin' awesome.

Mrs. Dude and the Dudettes? Simply the best. My brothers? Very cool. My extended family? Awesome folks. My friends? So much fun. My in-laws? Amazing.

And it goes on and on. I have an amazing support system and I would not have it any other way. But sadly, I have received hundreds of emails over the years asking for help. The number one issue? Family and friends dealing with their celiac disease, both the good and the bad.

For example:

My family doesn't understand and doesn't want to be educated about celiac disease. People die young in my family and wonder why. I love my family but they have actually gone as far as to tell me something was gluten-free that actually wasn't just "to see if I could tell". And that is just the half of it. I just don't know what to do. I don't know how to forgive them and I don't know if I can ever trust them again.

No excuse. Absolutely no excuse.

On the bright side, I have also received some heartwarming emails from those who have family that go out of their way.

Following are stories that will both inspire you and anger you. Now go hug someone who supports you.

Celiac Disease: It's All in the Family

I am doubly blessed when it comes to family life. I was raised in a pretty cool family with three older brothers and parents who held their act together just long enough to raise four respectable adults (and then completely fell to pieces). And now I am the husband of a woman who I love more than life itself and I get to raise two daughters of my own who I have watched in amazement as they have become young adults.

Yes…after growing up in a male-dominate household, I'm now surrounded by women and I wouldn't have it any other way. If you read my blog (bless your little hearts), you know them as Mrs. Dude and the Dudettes.

This is our celiac story.

In April of 2007, I was diagnosed with bladder cancer. The Dudettes were 11 and 8. While it was a major health scare and a huge "holy crap" moment in my life, thankfully it was not life-threatening so Mrs. Dude and I decided not to tell the kids that I had cancer because that word has such connotations attached to it. Whenever I came back from a procedure, we would just tell them that daddy has a few health issues and the doctors are making sure he's all better. The word "cancer" never entered our vocabulary with them. I suppose they'll find out when they read this article.

Just kidding…we told them a few years later.

When I was diagnosed with celiac disease six months later (yeah…good times…let's not even get started on my pulmonary embolisms in 2008), Mrs. Dude and I were thrown for a loss. We had never heard of the disease or the word gluten. You see, when you get diagnosed with celiac disease, the only instructions you receive from the doctor are, "Don't eat gluten ever again." And I'm thinking, "Uummm…ok…no problem. By the way, what the heck is gluten??"

It was a new world we were entering…one that seemed absolutely overwhelming. Not only did we need to learn what I could no longer eat, but we had to make sure I was safe in my own house. So Mrs. Dude did what she does best. She took complete control of the situation and kicked total booty. She immersed herself in learning everything she needed to know about this new constant in our life. Before you know it, I had my own counter in our kitchen; my own toaster; my own blue sponge to wash my dishes; my own set of pots and pans; my own cabinet for my food, my own silverware drawer and my own shelf in the fridge. If I was going to get glutened in my own house, it would not be due to carelessness.

Enter the Dudettes. How do we get two pre-teens to understand the seriousness of daddy's new illness? Upon my diagnosis, we sat them down and explained to them what celiac disease was and how I can't eat gluten anymore. We told them how important this was and that even a crumb could make me sick. And then we walked them around the kitchen and showed them all the new "gluten-free" labels placed throughout and that means those areas are off-limits to them. Then we explained all the new rules. For example, they couldn't put their hands directly in the ice bin anymore unless they had washed them first. They couldn't use my peanut butter for their sandwiches. They couldn't drink daddy's beer. (Just seeing if you're still paying attention.)

And you know what? They got it. They never blinked. And before long, it became the new normal. The transition was made easier because our family came together for a single cause of keeping me healthy. I know how lucky I am, as I have received so many disturbing emails from fellow celiacs whose families don't take the disease seriously. From the father who doesn't believe in celiac disease so he feeds his daughter gluten to the family of doctors who dismiss their sister's celiac disease because it's just a fad disease. Honestly…you can't make this stuff up.

The family support is so huge. I just don't know where I'd be without it.

Now…what is it like from the Dudettes' perspective? That's a darn good question. I asked both of my kids to write a little something for this article, describing what it's been like having a father with celiac disease. Here's what they said.

"

Dudette #1
"I was in middle school when I found out my dad had celiac disease. I remember going into school the next day and telling my friends my dad is allergic to glucose. *[Dude note: Gotta love it!]* At first it was a challenge. I had to adapt to all these new kitchen rules like "don't touch the top shelf of the fridge, that's dads shelf", or "wash your hands before you go on his computer". The hardest part of having a father with celiac is when he gets sick and all of these thoughts take over my mind worrying if I was the one who got him "glutened" this time. It's hard watching someone you love constantly feeling sick and run down so often, but my dad is the strongest man I know and doesn't let celiac take over his life."

"

"

Dudette #2
"I would be lying if I said having my dad being diagnosed with Celiac didn't change my lifestyle, but I would also be lying if I said all of those changes were negative. I'll be honest, it was difficult at first. It definitely affected the entire family. But despite the hard encounters my dad has been forced to face, things have gotten better. Not in the sense that he feels amazing 24/7, or even most of the time, just in the way that my family and I have become more aware overall. I

think the hardest part of living with someone who has celiac is just seeing them struggle daily. My dad being diagnosed with celiac definitely changed some aspects of my home life. Yet, he is still the same amazing person he was six years ago, in spite of all the horrors he went through. Celiac may have changed my family, but it didn't affect my love and appreciation for the man who has to live with it."

"

And now let's hear from the woman who keeps the Dude Ranch running like a fine-tuned engine. What impact has celiac disease had on her life?

"

Mrs. Dude
"The day my husband's diagnosis came in was the end of life as we knew it. I knew going forward, everything would change. And it did.

I will be honest, I mourned along with him. He mourned the loss of NY bagels, real pizza and a good IPA. I mourned the loss of our spontaneous way of living. No more just grabbing a drink and something to eat at that cute new place. Now it takes a ton more work, planning and research to be that cute spontaneous couple.

I had so many thoughts zoom through my head at once. How would we eat out? Socialize? Travel? How in the world could we keep him safe? The world was full of gluten at every turn. And cross contamination??? Are you kidding me??!! Grrrr!! I was overwhelmed!

It has been quite the journey. Not as simple as we were told. "Avoid gluten and you will feel better." Unfortunately this stubborn little autoimmune has a mind of its own. It angers me. It saddens me. This disease has robbed me of my best friend ALOT of the time. I never thought this would be my competition. My fun-loving, vivacious, intelligent husband turns into a cranky, severely exhausted, brain-fogged twit that also suffers physically (I will spare those unpleasant details). Did I mention cranky?

To sum things up, this is a crappy, unappreciated disease that has challenged me. I will fight it to the end. No one messes with my Dude and gets away with it!"

"

Like I said…I'm blessed with an amazing family!

I hope you are too.

No Spousal Support for Celiac? Find Another Spouse.

I belong to several celiac forums and help people out where I can. I cannot tell you the number of people who do not get support from their spouses when they get diagnosed with celiac disease. It is so sad. Here are some of the complaints I hear:

"My husband says I can have a little gluten…it's no big deal."

"My husband constantly contaminates my gluten-free butter."

"My husband says celiac is a media created disease."

So two questions:
1) Why does it always seem to be the husband who lacks the compassion? Actually, don't answer that…or if you do, be gentle.
2) What the #$%$%# are these people thinking??

Do the words "in sickness and in health" ring a bell??

When you first get the dreaded celiac diagnosis, it is absolutely overwhelming. You feel like your entire life has been overturned. And in a way, it has. Nothing will be like it once was. I still remember going grocery shopping the day after my diagnosis and all I kept thinking as I was going up and down the aisles was "I can't have that. I can't have that. I can't have that. I can't have that." It really sux.

But if I had to do it without Mrs. Dude's support? I cannot even imagine. Immediately, she immersed herself in education about the disease. She went out and bought separate utensils and pots and pans. She made part of the kitchen off limits to everyone but me. She labeled all of the drawers, counters, etc. "gluten-free" to remind the kids and our guests. But more than anything else, she just made me feel like I was not in this alone. And because of this, it's five years later, I'm (somewhat) healthy, I've never cheated and living gluten-free just feels "normal" now.

But this post is not about me. It's about YOU.

You need this type of support. If your spouse is not behind you 100%, dig deep and figure out why. It is a tough journey having celiac disease and it's one nobody should go through alone. But to go through it while somebody in your own home is fighting it? Total BS. No, I'm not really advocating leaving your spouse. Suggesting? Maybe. But advocating…no.

But if your spouse is indeed in denial, you need to find another support system. The celiac community is indeed a wonderful group of people. Immerse yourself with them and all of the sudden, you won't feel so alone.

Join Twitter and hashtag gluten and celiac.

Find a celiac support group in your area.

And by all means, feel free to ping me whenever you want. I may not be your spouse, but I'm not half bad.

7 Ways to Support a New Celiac

I just received an email from a follower (don't laugh…I have followers!) that reinforces why I started this blog. Here is part of what he said:

"

My wife is a celiac diagnosed about 2.5 months now. She really truly feels better reading your entries as she doesn't feel alone and others are experiencing the same things she is. Anyway, I was wondering if in one of your posts you can address the things a spouse can do to help a celiac. I am trying to get all resources and knowledge possible. But I'm sure I'm missing something. Maybe a top 5 list of things a spouse can do to help out would be great. Like in the beginning what you really needed that your spouse couldn't provide just due to not knowing or something.

"

Well, you asked for 5, but I'm feeling quite helpful today, so here are 7 ways to support somebody just diagnosed with celiac disease.

1. Be patient. You both are about to enter a whole new world. A world where gluten is now your enemy. Give yourself time. Time to mourn the loss of your old life. Time to learn all you need to know about your new life. Time to adjust. Don't expect to waltz into your gluten-free world without some bumps in the road.

2. Be strict. I remember the first few weeks after my diagnosis telling Mrs. Dude that I can't make any promises that I won't cheat. Well, she gave me the death stare and got her point across quite clearly. And I have never cheated...not even once. I'm not saying it has to fall on you to make sure your spouse doesn't cheat, but don't make it easy either. Never give your approval. Never encourage her to just "take a bite" of your pizza. And if you've got a death stare, now is the right time to bring it out.

3. Be educated. As your spouse is trying to digest the celiac diagnosis, it may be too much for her to learn all she needs to learn. Read, read and read some more about celiac disease and gluten. There is a wealth of information out there. Know as much as you can possibly know. Knowledge is power.

4. Be communicative. Talk about your fears (both of you...your life will also be quite affected). Talk about your anger. Talk about your future. Just talk.

5. Be organized. Read my lips...NO MORE GLUTEN. Help her get your house in order. Make sure she has her own space in the kitchen where she knows she will always be safe.

6. Be careful. Gluten is in a lot of food. And just because it's not in a food item one day, it doesn't mean it won't be another day. Be your spouse's best advocate. Know what she can and can't have. Read ingredients for her. Look things up on Google for her. Yep, having celiac disease affects more than just the patient.

7. Be there. She will need you now more than ever. Don't let her down.

"I Never Thought" by Mrs. Dude

I thought I'd have Mrs. Dude handle the duties for this one and give the scoop of what it's truly like living with a celiac. Mrs. Dude, take it away.

————

I never thought I would hear myself say "DON'T KISS ME. I JUST ATE A BAGEL!"

I never thought I would worry about what color sponge my kids use (on that rare occasion when they wash the dishes.)

I never thought that once my kids outgrew the diaper bag years, I'd have to pack one for my husband (for food…not diapers).

I never thought I would be the hostess that would tackle my guests before they reached into the icemaker without using the scooper.

I never thought I'd use the word "contaminate" so much.

I never thought I would spend so much time hating a tiny little protein that you can't even see but still makes Gluten Boy sick!

I never thought I'd have to dissect the previous nine meals we ate when he doesn't feel well.

I never thought I would become the supermarket whore that I have become. I bop from one to another without looking back!

I never thought we would be the ones that food servers cringe at.

I never thought I would need my reading glasses to food shop!

I never thought Google would become such an imperative ingredient in my cooking.

I never thought I'd get so mad when the Dude emptied the dishwasher this week and put "his" cutting board in the girl's bread drawer.

I never thought I'd have to worry about the dogs licking his face (our dogs are NOT gluten-free).

I never thought I'd be married to someone with the nickname "Dude".

I never thought I would come to respect a group of people I have never met as much as I respect the celiac community.

I never thought I would say this, but my gluten boy has really turned into Gluten Dude. I love what his voice/rants have added to the celiac community. He is passionate about everything in life (which can be exhausting…good thing he doesn't have a blog about politics!!)

A Gut-Wrenching Love Note from a Mom to her 8-Year-Old Celiac Daughter

The following note, which was sent to me privately and posted with the Mom's permission, needs no introduction. Please just read it and share it. This is the side of celiac disease the public eye does not see. And we need them to see it.

"

Hi Gluten Dude. I write my 8 year old daughter love notes to an email account I set up for her as a baby. Over the last year and a half thru Hell – diagnosing and treating her celiac – I have penned many a letter. When she's older, perhaps a mother herself, I will give her access. This last month has been filled with excruciating pain and frustration for her.

This is last night's letter:

Sometimes at night, after you've gone to sleep, I crawl into bed with you and wrap you in my arms. It is only when you are fast asleep, that I can take off my armor, put away my cape, and put down my guard.

It is then, that my tears find yours on the pillow.

When you look at me, with eyes filled with terror, exclaiming, "Mommy! I'm scared about what's happening in my body!" and melt into my arms, I too am scared. I'm horrified. But I cannot tell you that. I need to be strong for you. In my heart though, I'm crying right along beside you. Every single tear.

It's only after you've cried yourself to sleep in pain, that I can cry with you.

I put my hand upon your swollen belly, as if I truly had Super Mommy Powers, and that I can magically draw out what ails you. I envision your pain, passing thru my hand, up my arm, and into my own belly. I can take it. Just give it to me. Oh, how I beg, God, just give it to me. Please. I'll do anything. Please.

I'm sad. I'm mad. I'm pissed off. I'm scared. I'm helpless.

I am all those things, and more. Most importantly, I am your mother. I will never give up on you. I will fight every last battle, right along your side. You might be small, you might be scared, but you are strong. Whatever this latest challenge, you will be OK. You will. There are no other alternatives.

I wish I had the answers to your questions. I wish I could wipe it all away. I wish I could love you all better. If love was the answer, you'd be healed, for my love for you is limitless, and eternal.

You are my sweetest angel, and I don't know why someone as kind hearted and loving as you, is faced with such challenges. You're too young to struggle so much. Now I truly grasp the concept of "not fair".

But what you are not…is alone. You might feel that no one understands what you're going through, and no, I don't know what it's like to be so sick at 7 and then 8. But what I do know, is that with all my heart and soul, you are my daughter, and when you're in pain, I am too. I just can't show you.

When you were born, I gave you a piece of my heart, and my heart breaks for you now. Now I will crawl into my own bed, put my head on my own pillow, and I will not cry any more tears tonight, but you will never leave my thoughts and prayers.

There is not a day that goes by, that I don't wish upon a star, that this will all pass, and you can go back to being a kid.

Maybe tonight my wish will come true.

"

201

Is Semen Gluten-Free?

Dude note: If you are offended by risqué innuendos (all done in humor), you may want to pass on this one. If you want to be entertained, or actually want to know the answer, read on.

Yes…I just went there.

No…I am not curious for my own behalf (not that there's anything wrong with it).

The request came from somebody on my Facebook page. Her name is…oh wait…I probably shouldn't share her name.

Anyway, here is how the conversation went:

Her: I thought you'd be the best person to ask this "seriously want to keep anonymous" question…no offense. Gross but a concern for us Celiac gals…has anyone ever tested sperm for gluten? For once, Google can't seem to help me! Thanks, I have always wanted to know and who in the world could I ask but you.

Me: I'll take that as a backhanded compliment (lol).

Her: No offense meant; just don't know of anyone with Celiac that tells it like you do and would even answer the request without thinking I'm a perv…it was a total compliment! Believe me, I brought it up once online with a Celiac friend and I thought she was going to choke on her tongue due to the stuttering!

I told her it was a tough JOB but I was totally UP for the challenge.

After spending some time online, I couldn't find a definitive answer. And I thought…this really BLOWS.

So I looked some more (and came across some disturbing websites along the way…which I've bookmarked) and still nothing. This totally SUCKS.

So I decided to SWALLOW my pride and ask around a bit.

Ok...I'll stop with the innuendos now.

Here are the ingredients of a typical batch: fructose sugar, water, ascorbic acid, citric acid, enzymes, protein, phosphate and bicarbonate buffers and zinc.

Mmmm...mmmm...good.

But is it safe?

Sure looks gluten-free to me but I still could not find anyone to confirm my belief. And nobody volunteered to do a taste test.

But then I finally found what I was looking for. The Celiac Disease Center in Chicago confirmed that we can all rest easy.

No...there is no gluten in semen.

Bottoms up!

How to Survive Being a Friend of a Celiac

Let me introduce you to David Z, a very good friend of mine. We had him and his wife over for drinks a few nights ago, and he said it would be interesting to view celiac disease from a friend's perspective. I thought it was brilliant and he had the below post in my inbox by 6 the next morning.

How to Survive Being a Friend of a Celiac Sufferer

The above title of this blog post is not accurate. I know, strange way to open a blog entry, but it's true. Allow to me explain.

Being a friend of Gluten Dude I remember quite distinctly the first time we engaged socially after he was diagnosed. Dude had let us known that he would like us to come over for drinks and snacks and after a few he regaled us with his journey through celiac. I was both mesmerized and a bit sad. My friend of all these years was afflicted with this insidious disease that could attack at any moment, brought on by a mere crumb or fallen morsel.

As he educated us, my mind interpreted his restrictions as a confinement of the pleasures of life and I left that night being both bonded with my friend but simultaneously pitying him.

As good friends, we wanted to reciprocate the invite so we invited Dude and Mrs. Dude over to our house for drinks and snacks. My wife took great pains to try to purchase foods that were marked gluten-free and laid out a spread.

Unfortunately more than 70% of the food we put out was too questionable for Gluten Dude to partake in so all night he ate carrots and rice crackers, which to me tasted like packing peanuts. More pity for my friend, and a feeling of hopelessness that we would never be able to break Dude from the confines of his "house imprisonment" and his world of gluten-free that he had created under his own roof.

But over the next few months, and the more we 'hung' with Gluten Dude, something interesting happened.

We consciously or subconsciously, not sure which, stopped trying so hard. We stopped trying to OVER-research foods and restaurants that would be appropriate for Dude. We stopped agonizing over which house we would be going over to or how Dude might feel if all he had to eat was carrots.

But most of all, I stopped thinking of Dude as my friend with Celiac and instead went back to thinking of him as my friend...someone that makes our lives better for knowing.

I also realized that although Celiac is an important cause for him, it didn't define who the Dude was. HE defined himself.

With that relaxed state of mind we invited The Dudes over for our annual Halloween Party. Quite casually we set up a Gluten free station with the foods we knew the Dude could enjoy. In doing so we created an environment where Dude could sit back and enjoy the party and put Celiac worries on hold for a night. It was special for us. Special because our good friend could be our good friend, and not the man I originally pitied.

As I write this I fondly think back to just last night where we partook of Friday night drinks and snacks at the Dude's house. It was the usual fair of crazy drinks and snacks, generously passed out by G. Dude. But they have long ago ceased to be Gluten Free snacks and have just become snacks...just as my good friend ceased to be a celiac sufferer and has just become my friend.

Being a friend of a someone with celiac is not about surviving the friendship, it is about thriving and celebrating who the person is and the value they create in your life.

My Letter to the Parents of a Depressed Girl with Celiac Disease

Dear Mom & Dad,

You don't know me, but I know your daughter. She's not in a good place and you don't seem to care. How do I know this? Because she reached out to me a few days ago privately.

You see…I'm a celiac and I try to help my fellow celiacs as much as humanly possible. So the other day, I posted a picture of my blue sponge on my Facebook page. My blue sponge is used specifically for my gluten-free cookware that does not go in the dishwasher. This is to help prevent cross-contamination, which helps keep me safe.

There was a lot of great back and forth during the course of the day. But then I got the following private message from your daughter.

> "
>
> Your picture of your blue sponge and comments from people made me upset. Here at home, I have to make my food in my room. I had my own gluten-free bench and cookware but everyone went out of their way to use it so I had to stop. My family makes fun of me for it. I've been sick for almost 2 years since my celiac started, yet my family thinks it's not important. I'm jealous of people who have safe kitchens with kind and caring families. End of rant. I'm going to make my lunch…in my bedroom…again.
>
> Thank you.
> From a depressed celiac.
>
> "

This is your daughter speaking…and she's telling me how you make fun of her for her disease. I was angry. I was frustrated. I was so sad for her. I really wanted to dig a little to find out what could possibly cause a family to be so callous. So I reached out to her with the following response.

I'm so sorry [name retracted]. Can you tell me a bit about your family and why you think they don't take your celiac seriously?

Here is what she said:

I know why. Just after I got sick, my brother, his girlfriend and baby moved in with us. At the time, I was in hospital a few times. I spent 2 months in bed being sick. I couldn't do anything. My family hated it that I wouldn't look after the baby. I lost 30 kg, threw up every half an hour and I couldn't eat for days at a time. So basically my family turned their back on me.

When I started eating small amounts of food, they gave me my bench but behind my back used it all the time. My family was there when I had to have cancer tests and they were told how important it was that I be careful of even the most tiny bit of gluten. Still didn't care. They just hate me cause I got sick and had to put myself first for a change. Health always comes first.

So there you have it. Your daughter thinks you hate her. And why? Because she has a disease that has ONE treatment only and you are making it impossible for her to stay healthy.

Since I'm only getting one side of the story, I won't go in full attack mode here folks. But I implore you. Do some research. Learn the facts about celiac disease. Untreated celiac disease can get ugly. How ugly?

Untreated celiac disease can be life threatening. Celiacs are more likely to be afflicted with problems relating to malabsorption, including osteoporosis, tooth enamel defects, central and peripheral nervous system disease, pancreatic disease, internal hemorrhaging, organ disorders (gall bladder, liver, and spleen), and gynecological disorders. Untreated celiac disease has also been linked an increased risk of certain types of cancer, especially intestinal lymphoma. There are no drugs to treat celiac disease and there is no cure. But celiacs can lead normal, healthy lives by following a gluten-free diet. This means avoiding all products derived from wheat, rye, and barley. (source: MassGeneral Hospital)

You got that? No drugs. No cure. And untreated can result in cancer.

That is celiac disease. It's not a fad. It's not a joke. It's not a minor food allergy. It's a disease.

If you have any questions about keeping your daughter safe, please contact me. I'm here to help.

In the meantime, please take care of her. When someone reaches out to a complete stranger about her family, you know she's in a bad place. Get her back in a good place. As her parents, that's your job.

Sincerely,

Gluten Dude

What Do You Do When Your In-laws Won't Feed You?

Let me ask you a question. During the holidays, did you eat any meals at someone else's house? And if so, were you treated like crap? Did you feel like an outcast because of your food restrictions? If not, awesome. You have true friends and family. If so, I'm sorry. It looks like you're not alone.

I received the following message after a holiday weekend:

> "
>
> Hi Gluten Dude. I just recently came across your page. I have a question for you about gluten etiquette I guess lol. For the past two years I have not eaten gluten; every time we go to my mother-in-law's house, whether it be Christmas, Thanksgiving, etc., she has absolutely nothing to offer me for food.
>
> I have to sit there and watch my husband eat. My sister has gone gluten-free in the past year and she deals with it with her husband's family also.
>
> Are we expecting too much that our family members would have at least one thing to offer us? From our standpoint we would never have somebody come to our house and not have something for them to eat .
>
> I would ask or look it up online but to us it just seems that they obviously don't care enough to try to have something.
>
> What is your whole take on that situation?
>
> "

Oh boy, do I have a take on this. *First, I'll be gentle Dude.*

I'm so sorry you have to experience this. Do I find it absolutely ridiculous that your own family can't prepare something for you? Absolutely. Actually, ridiculous is being too kind. I find it rude, ill-mannered and just totally crappy.

So much for gentle Dude.

Who has family over and not have something for them to eat?? And don't tell me it's too difficult to prepare a safe meal. I've said it before and I'll say it again: It ain't rocket science folks. There's this thing called the internet where if you WANT TO LEARN how to keep a celiac safe, you can look it up.

But that's the key: you need to WANT TO LEARN. If you can have your family over and simply watch your daughter-in-law not eat, well…that doesn't say a whole lot about you, now does it?

I do have a quick solution for you. If you know they are not going to make anything for you, bring your own food. Problem solved.

I gotta ask…what exactly is your husband's take on this? He's the one who should be taking the issue up with his parents. Is he really willing to sit there and eat dinner while you aren't eating anything?

My suggestion is that you open the lines of communication. Maybe your in-laws don't believe in the whole gluten-free thing for whatever reason. Maybe they do and just feel too overwhelmed by it. You will never know unless you talk openly with them.

There's that word again: communication. I'm telling ya folks…it's the key to fixing life's problems.

Sorry for the tough love. It comes from the heart.

A Mom 'Protects' Her Celiac Daughter by Hiding Her Diagnosis

No. Words.

There was an article in the Washington Post written by a mom whose daughter had just been diagnosed with a severe peanut allergy. And because the mom wanted her daughter to be happy for as long as possible, she hid the diagnosis from her for several weeks, allowing her to eat as many peanuts as she wanted during that time.

Incredible, right?

Except it didn't happen that way. The "healthy" daughter was actually diagnosed with celiac disease and the mom fed her gluten for several weeks because SHE was the one who couldn't handle the diagnosis.

The strangest thing about this? She seems proud of herself. Why else would she write an article about it for one of the largest newspapers in the country? Meaning she fully admitted to having a very crappy parenting moment to the entire nation. Who does that? As I was reading the article, I kept waiting for the AHA moment where she has some self-reflection. Nope. Instead, we got these gems:

She was happy, largely asymptomatic and growing like a weed. I worried that the burden of knowing about her condition might do more harm than good.

Dude note: Really? No immediate worries about her insides being attacked by her own body and being ripped apart? Ok then.

My friend casually suggested that I consider cutting gluten from her diet. Normally I would dismiss the idea but I opened my big mouth and raised this topic with my daughter's endocrinologist a few days later and the whole diagnostic process was set in motion.

Dude note: You consider trying to help your daughter "opening your big mouth". Hmmm...I consider it...parenting.

It was my daughter's gastrointestinal system we were talking about, yet it was me that felt punched in the gut.

Dude note: Your 11 year old daughter just got diagnosed with a serious autoimmune disease and all you thought about was how it affected YOU? Mom of the Year you ain't.

Countless well-meaning people tried to console me. I appreciated people's kindness but the truth was, I didn't want to deal with it.

Dude note: Ahh...denial. I think they teach that the first week in Parenting 101. I must have missed classes that week.

My husband runs an association of gastroenterologists and I told him, "I want you to search far and wide and find me a doctor who says we can blow this off. Our child is perfectly healthy and asymptomatic."

Dude note: [mouth wide open...trying to get words out...]

I had no such luck. They told us that while children with celiac who eat gluten can appear to be fine, doing so continuously can cause damage in the longer-term that has been linked to an increased risk of intestinal cancers, osteoporosis, and infrequently neurological conditions like epilepsy.

Dude note: Yay...she saw the light!

Still, we held off telling her while she was away at sleep-away camp to give her a few more carefree weeks. We told ourselves we'd tell her when she came home and we went on our beach vacation. That didn't happen. The days flew by and we all indulged in a gluttonous gluten-fest and she never asked about the biopsy results.

Dude note: So much for the light.

Finally, driving home from the beach — several weeks after my husband and I knew about the diagnosis — she finally asked. "Do you really want to know?" I asked her.

Dude note: Are you effing kidding me!? "Do you really want to know?" Does it matter what she wants?? TELL HER. Yes...I was actually screaming at my monitor. And what if she said no? Would you have not told her and kept up the charade?

We agreed to learn about the disease together, gently dip our toe into the celiac waters and gradually make the switch to a gluten-free diet. And that's what we did.

Dude note: So you "gradually" made the switch to gluten-free? Knowing full well that every bite of gluten was poison to her body? Again...I. Have. No. Words.

So here's my question to the community. Why? Why would any parent feed their kid gluten after a celiac diagnosis? Is it because gluten-free is a fad (that can't die soon enough)? Is it because those who eat gluten-free are the butt end of a barrage of jokes on TV? Is it because the conversation seems to be always about the food...and never about the disease? Maybe. Maybe not. Maybe this is actually an amazing mom who just had a 3 week brain fart. Who knows?

All I know is if the diagnosis was cancer, diabetes, a peanut allergy or a laundry list of other diseases, I would assume she would have started the treatment immediately.

But celiac? Nah...we can wait a while. After all, I need to protect my daughter.

Dude, My Girlfriend has Celiac and Cheats. What Do I Do?

I was laying bed last night at the ungodly hour of 3am wide awake. After another brutally long work day, my mind was simply too wired to fall into a slumber. I learned a trick many years ago if you have having trouble falling asleep. You try to find five different sounds that you hear. In the still of the night, not an easy task. The idea is that your mind will stop racing, which will help you fall into a relaxed state.

So I gave it a shot. And you know what I heard? Silence. Utter silence. Sure…occasionally one of my pups would snore or Mrs. Dude would scream out how much she loves me in her sleep, but I couldn't get to the five sounds. And then it came to me. The lack of sound wasn't silence. It was peace. It was tranquility. It was gratefulness.

There is no war outside my bedroom. My family is not going to bed hungry. There are no riots in the streets. I have a home. I have friends. Dang…I'm a pretty lucky guy. And with that…I fell asleep.

What does this have to do with celiac? It's a stretch, but there's a connection. Here is an email I received recently:

> "
>
> Hi Gluten Dude:
>
> I have a good friend who is a bartender. She has Celiac Disease. She continues to drink craft beer. What are the long-term ramifications of this behavior? The rest of her diet is gluten-free from what I can tell. I'm talking more than 3 beers & sometimes it's way more at least 3-4 times a week. What should I do as a friend? My experience with celiac is limited, but I have been reviewing articles & see some of the

side-effects associated with consuming gluten in her. What happens if she doesn't stop this behavior? Is it going to kill her? Or just make her life uncomfortable? Thank you for your time & website.

"

Here's the deal. Who knows what will happen if she keeps cheating on her celiac disease. She may develop intestinal or stomach cancer and die an awful (and unnecessary) death. Or maybe lymphoma.

Researchers at Columbia University announced in 2013 that patients with celiac disease who had persistent intestine damage (identified with repeat biopsy) had a higher risk of lymphoma than patients whose intestines healed. The study shows that "celiac patients with persistent villous atrophy-as seen on follow-up biopsy-have an increased risk of lymphoma, while those with healed intestines have a risk that is significantly lower, approaching that of the general population."

Or she may live for another 60 years, but I guarantee it won't be a fruitful 60 years.

So those are the "health-related" reasons why she should stop. Now here is my personal opinion. If she's drinking 3-4 beers almost every night, the issue may go beyond celiac. I bartended for many years back in my youth, and I've seen some bartenders who couldn't handle being behind the bar without partaking in the spirits that surrounded them. It ain't pretty.

But it goes deeper than that…and now I'll finally swing back to how the heck this relates to my dream. If you are a celiac and you cheat…you're weak. If you are a celiac, feel like crap a lot and yet you eat really unhealthy food…you're weak. If you're more concerned with being normal than being healthy…you're weak.

And yeah…we all have weak moments, but instead of being weak, be grateful. If celiac is the biggest issue in your life, then you've got a pretty good life. And if you are going to cast that aside just because you want to drink craft beer, there is nothing I can do to change your mind.

Find that tranquility. That inner peace. That silence. And sleep like a baby tonight.

What Do You Do When Your Husband is Pretty Much an A**wipe?

Oh boy. Oh boy, oh boy, oh boy. This one is just plain old ugly. We've all heard the stories about family members not taking gluten-free seriously. Even spouses. Makes me thank my lucky stars (again and again and again) for Mrs. Dude.

But this guy goes above and beyond in his assholishness and our gluten-free friend is asking for advice. It's time for some tough love...for both of them.

Here's the email I received:

> "
>
> Hey Gluten Dude. When I was first diagnosed as gluten intolerant through a genetic blood test, my husband refused to believe it meant anything would be different. Now here we are, 5 years later. And he STILL says, "You are overreacting. You are not celiac and a little gluten won't hurt you."
>
> Of all people, the one who has watched me be sick after contamination; the one who knows how terrified I am to eat at any restaurant (I have been glutened by a restaurant with a gluten-free menu); he still doesn't get it.
>
> I have color-coded everything in my kitchen with RED being my "don't use this for gluten" code. Still, he eats pizza, from the kitchen counter, wiping his bearded and mustached mouth with my RED dish towels. Served off of my granite counter top. Reheated in my toaster oven or on the turntable in the microwave.
>
> I finally blew my top when I pointed out that he was using a red towel or utensil or wire mesh strainer marked RED to strain his

217

bow-tie pasta and he dismissed my complaint with his usual "It won't hurt you. You are overreacting. You are not celiac."

His carelessness makes me afraid to use my own kitchen without first washing everything and drying with a fresh out of the dryer red towel. Every meal. If I get contaminated, the distress begins between 20 and 40 minutes and continues for 4 to 6 hours. This makes me afraid to eat. Even in my own home because of the chance of cross-contamination.

When even the people closest to you don't understand and don't respect this disease, I lose heart of ever healing. Since my blow up, my husband has made an effort to keep my red coded items separate in the kitchen, but still treats me as if I am "nagging" when I find him using them with gluten products. I need a kosher kitchen. Not to separate dairy and meat. But to isolate gluten from my gluten-free zones!

”

Ok...like I said; tough love time.

First...to the woman who wrote the email. Have you been tested for celiac? The reason I ask is that there is no valid blood test to diagnose gluten intolerance, as far as I know. Have you been to a legit doctor and been tested for celiac with blood work and an endoscopy? Not that I am remotely excusing your husband's boor-like behavior, but since it seems you are going to stick it out with him and his lame point seems only to be "you don't have celiac disease", perhaps a diagnosis will turn him back into a human being again.

5 years? That's a long time. You're more patient than I would be.

Now…to the husband. You seriously wipe your beard and mustache using a dish towel?? Forget if it's red, blue, paisley or plaid? Ever hear of a napkin? Look, whether you "believe" in gluten intolerance or not, didn't you take some vows some years back? Remember the sentence "for better or for worse, in sickness and in health"? Ring a bell at all? Dude, she already feels like shit that she has to go through the ringer to try to keep her home safe and stay healthy. Don't make her feel even worse about it. She's not asking you to eat gluten-free in the house. Just to respect her space, respect her wishes and respect her as a person.

If you can't do that…gluten is the least of your marriage's problems.

Chapter 7: OMG!! Can I Still Drink??

I know. I know. It's such a shallow question. I mean, you've got celiac disease. Alcohol is the last thing on your mind. Or is it??

I've been known to enjoy a cocktail or two and for me, it was front and center in my mind. Ok...fine...I was in pure panic mode. Can I drink beer? What about wine...or vodka...or gin...or bourbon...or (oh please say yes) my special margarita (lots of fresh lime, dash of orange juice)?????

Rest easy. You can still drink. But you gotta be careful because there is a minefield of BAD INFORMATION out there. Both telling you something is safe when it's not and telling you something is dangerous when it's not. Yeah...typical of our disease.

Stick with me kid and I'll show the way.

Cheers!!

The Ultimate Guide to Gluten-Free Alcohol

Here's the latest news. This article is about booze. If it's not what you choose, for you this may be a snooze. But if you like your brews during the holiday woo-hoos, you may be confused as to what booze you can infuse and which ones you must refuse. No need to get the blues. Stick with me…you've got nothing to lose.

Ok…that was exhausting to write.

If you are at a celiac support group or have an online following, I have a great way to cause some controversy. Simply say "[insert any liquor here] is gluten-free." You will certainly get your share of opinions, some of them spot on, some of them fear-based and some of them just totally bizarre.

I will try to set you as straight as humanly possible. But alcohol is one of those issues where I always say LISTEN TO YOUR BODY. And there are still some question marks regarding specific alcohol.

Ok…ready for some fun? Here we go.

BEER

Beer is split into two camps: Gluten-free and Gluten-removed. This is pretty simple. Well, let me rephrase that. This "should" be pretty simple, but alas it's actually very complicated.

Gluten-free beer is just that. Totally gluten-free and completely safe.

Gluten-removed beer is actually made with gluten, but then, so they say, the gluten is removed using a proprietary process, making it fall below 20ppm. I don't drink these and I never will. Naturally, they market themselves as gluten-free, even though technically they're not allowed to.

You want ever more confusion? The CSA, a top celiac organization, gave their seal of approval to Omission, a gluten-removed beer, even though their seal implicitly states that "our Seal Program does not allow the use of oats or ingredients that are derived from gluten-containing grains that have been refined in such a way to remove the gluten."

How's that for a contradiction?

And let's add one more layer of confusion into the mix. Some standard beers actually say they are safe for celiacs, falling under the 20ppm. These are not gluten-removed beers but beers actually containing gluten. Yeah…crazy I know.

Here is what one major brewer, Heineken, says on their website's FAQ page for the question "Does your beer contain gluten?

"Beer contains gluten, which comes from the grain used to brew it. Only a fraction of the gluten in the grain gets into the beer – the exact amount depends on the kind of grain used. Brewing beer with barley leaves only traces of gluten in the beer, while wheat contributes considerably more. The brewing process can also affect gluten content. Generally speaking, the clearer and blonder the beer is, the less gluten it contains. Some people are allergic to gluten and have to follow a diet that minimizes or excludes their gluten intake. Whether beer can be part of such a diet or not depends on the extent of the allergy and the type of beer consumed. In many cases, lager beers pose no problem for people who have a gluten allergy. However, it is up to individuals to assess their own sensitivity."

I think I speak for the gluten-free community when I say…HUH?

My personal favorites: Glutenberg (especially the IPA), Pyro, Groundbreaker, Ghostfish

Oh…and though I'm not a cider kind of guy, there are lots of gluten-free ciders on the market too.

Phew…moving on.

VODKA, GIN, RUM, TEQUILA

As long as they are non-flavored, they are safe. Yes, I know some of them are made with wheat. But the distillation process removes all gluten, leaving them with a whole lot of goodness behind. And if you want to be extra careful with the vodka, there are plenty made from corn, grape or potato.

Yes…I know there are still many celiacs who swear these items are not gluten-free. But science says otherwise. And so does The University of Chicago Celiac Disease Center. They say that *"in pure spirits, the distillation process makes these beverages safe because the protein is removed. However, flavored spirits may contain malt, and should be avoided."*

And by the way, if you're wondering why removing the gluten from liquor is ok but removing it from beer is not, that's a valid question. And here's a valid answer: It's a totally different process. Science proves that the distillation process of hard liquor removes all gluten. The process that gluten-removed beer uses is not distillation at all. They use enzymes, etc. It's proprietary and unproven.

My personal favorites:

- Vodka: Titos

- Gin: Hendricks, Bombay Sapphire East

- Rum: Not a big fan, but I'll drink a Dark and Stormy every blue moon

- Tequila: Casamigos (amazing!!), Don Julio, Cabo Wabo. If making margaritas, just stick with good old Cuervo Gold

SCOTCH, BOURBON, WHISKEY, RYE

My dad would enjoy one scotch (or two or three) every night after work. This eventually led to his downfall and way-too-early death. Perhaps subconsciously that's why I don't drink it. Or maybe it's just because I hate the taste.

Anyway, my research says these are all gluten-free. But I have heard many, many varying viewpoints from my fellow celiacs about these items. Here's a sampling of responses I received after posting that whiskey's, etc. are gluten-free:

"You are spreading mis-information! Some whiskeys, bourbons and scotches are aged in barrels coated in wheat paste. Very sensitive celiacs can react!"

"Dude, sorry but you are misinformed. You are correct about the science of distillation removing gluten, but I've never met a distiller that doesn't add the mash back into their final product. They all do it but most will tell you they don't."

"Wait – I read from multiple sources that whiskey, scotch and bourbon aren't gluten-free!"

"I hate to tell you, Gluten Dude, but i am celiac and i cannot drink those liquors."

I'll tell you…being a celiac can be exhausting. Here is what I say to the people above: Perhaps you are sensitive to something else in these liquors and it has nothing to do with gluten. Perhaps not. I reached out to a few popular distillers and heard nothing but crickets in response. I've said it before and I'll say it again. LISTEN TO YOUR BODIES.

WINE

Wine is gluten-free. And you can ignore the rumors about the barrels being sealed with wheat paste. Wine is fine. Especially when you dine. Just don't take mine. And don't drink nine. Ok, that's my last line.

My personal favorites: Red, White & Rose.

So there you have it.

Oh wait…one more item. Since my celiac diagnosis, my tolerance level has seem to gone down some. If you are going to imbibe, be careful and drink lots of water during the course of the evening.

Stay thirsty my friends.

The Gluten-Free Beer Wars: Health vs Profit

Gluten-free Beer vs Gluten-removed Beer
Safe Grains vs Barley
Groundbreaker vs Omission
Health vs Profit

There was a very, very interesting article recently on the current state of gluten-free beer. And more specifically, on Omission beer's fight with the FDA to be able to label itself "Gluten Free".

Here's a quick recap on Omission Beer. Instead of using gluten-free grains to brew their beer, they use barley, a big celiac no-no, and then remove the gluten using a proprietary technique so it falls below the 20ppm threshold. Their method produces a more traditional tasting beer (so they say). But scientists say it leaves tiny gluten fragments behind and that it may not be safe for those with celiac disease. And recent tests done in Canada on other "gluten-removed" beer found gluten in these beers too.

Because Omission is made with gluten, they cannot label it gluten-free in the United States. It also must carry a warning that no tests exist to verify gluten in beer, at least until the FDA rules on the issue. The bureau ruled last May that affixing a "gluten-free" label to a product made with barley, rye, wheat or crossbreeds would be "inherently misleading."

(Ironically, they can label it gluten-free in Denmark, Canada and within Oregon, where the beer is brewed. I've said it before and I'll say it again…our labeling laws just suck.)

What is Omission Beer's response to all of this? They say, and I quote, *"There's no denial that we're going to find pieces of protein [gluten] in the beer. Those don't go away. But those pieces are small. That's our view on it."*

When I wrote about Omission Beer in the past, it quickly became a hot topic of discussion, generating over 150 comments. The verdict seems that most celiacs who take their health seriously will not risk it. And many of the ones who did came to regret it. Now Craft Brew Alliance, who brews Omission Beer, is lobbying Congress to push the FDA to allow them to label their beer gluten-free. Here's a blurb from the article which states it quite eloquently:

Craft Brew's full-court press leaves federal regulators balancing the health of a small number of consumers against the moneymaking interests of a politically connected business. In this case, the health of 3 million people with celiac hang in the balance with the nation's ninth-largest brewer fighting to maintain $160 million in annual sales in an increasingly competitive beer market.

Now of course, Congress has gotten itself involved. Oh joy. Note dripping sarcasm. Five congressmen, naturally all from the Northwest where Craft Brew Alliance is located, sent the FDA a letter saying they were being "unnecessarily rigid". That's right folks...keeping celiacs safe is unnecessarily rigid. How dare the FDA worry about our health when there are profits to be made?!

Here is what I want: transparency and honesty. I know, when it comes to big business and the government, I'm kidding myself. The fact is I've heard from many of my fellow celiacs who have tried Omission or Daura. Almost all of them say "never again." There is enough evidence that these gluten-removed beers pose a risk to those who cannot tolerate gluten. So there is no way in hell they should be able to label themselves gluten-free.

Here is what I say to these brewers: If you want to make a gluten-free beer, then make a damn GLUTEN FREE beer. Rise to the challenge. Be creative. Don't try to change the laws at my community's expense so you can make more money.

Other companies are managing to make truly gluten-free beers that taste just fine. There is a microbrewery called Ground Breaker that makes the most amazing gluten-free beer. They make an IPA, a pale, a dark and an experimental ale. And they make their beers in a dedicated gluten-free facility, more than I can say for the folks at Omission.

While Omission beer is willing to accept that their beer is making some celiacs sick, James Neumeister, the owner of Ground Breaker, says that if he heard that gluten-intolerant drinkers were having unpleasant reactions to his beer, *"I'd have to be committed. I'd be a nervous wreck."*

How about that? A company with a conscience.

That's who I want making my beer.

Don't Fear the Beer!

2017 Gluten Dude: Since I wrote this post, New Planet now makes gluten-REMOVED beer as well. I no longer support them. But at the time, it was the first decent gfree beer I tasted. Ok…carry on.

Let me be clear.
I really like beer.
In 2007, I truly did fear
A life without beer.

Red Bridge was here.
But it wasn't good beer.
Bards then drew near.
One taste and…oh dear.

Then a whisper in my ear
"New Planet tastes like beer."
What did I just hear?
Was it really sincere?

"A true gluten-free beer!!"
I let out a cheer.
I shed a big tear
Then swung on my chandelier.

Then Groundbreaker Beer
Found its way here.
Who created this beer?
A gluten-free beer engineer?

Glutenberg then appeared.
After I paid the cashier.

I said "It's a new frontier
In gluten-free beer."

Omission and Daura, being quite cavalier,
Call themselves gluten-free beer.
They're not gluten-free beers.
And they can both kiss my rear.

Last week a new beer
Suddenly appeared.
It was gluten-FREE beer.
To drink it I volunteered.

Now let me be clear
And I'm being sincere.
Pyro is the beer of the year
For gluten-free beers.

They are another pioneer
In gluten-free beer.
I could make a career
From drinking their beer.

This beer should be revered
Just like Britney Spears
In her glory years
(Before she grabbed the shears).

The bottom line here
Is don't fear the beer.
Real gluten-free beer is here
And to that...I SAY CHEERS!

Chapter 8: Celebrities and Celiac: The Good, the Bad and the Ugly

I know we've done some heavy duty lifting up to this point, so let's try to end this book on a bit of a lighter note. Let's talk some celebrity juice.

I covered some celebs over the years. Oh boy have I covered them. Some great (i.e. Jennifer Esposito) and some downright appalling (i.e. Dr. Oz).

Heck, my Kim Kardashian rant sort of put me on the map.

Have they helped or hurt our cause? Well, I wrote a lot about them early in my blogging years when they were either jumping on the bandwagon or making fun of us. But not so much in the past few years.

And that my friends is progress. Enjoy.

Dear Gwyneth: Please Shut Up

> 2017 Gluten Dude: Ms. Paltrow was one of the first celebs to jump on the gluten-free bandwagon. But my god, was she annoying about it and didn't quite have all of her facts straight. Shocking…I know. Anyway, this post goes back to 2011. She's been pretty quiet lately. Cheers to that.

Dear Gwyneth:

I know your intentions are good. But you and your Hollywood friends are really doing those with celiac disease a huge disservice. Going gluten-free is not a "diet choice" for us. It is not "key to losing weight" as you say. It's not the South Beach Diet or any of those other ridiculous fad diets out there that promise a shortcut to a healthy body and soul.

You want to be healthy? Eat smart, eat less and exercise a lot. It's been this way since the beginning of time and it will never, ever change.

Four years ago when I was diagnosed with celiac disease, most had not heard of the disease and had no idea what gluten was (me included). So if I was eating out, I needed to be very specific in my ordering because it was such an unknown to the general public. And because of that, I was taken very seriously. Chefs came out to speak with me. Waitresses asked a thousand questions to make sure I wouldn't get sick. And while it was, and continues to be, a huge pain in the ass, it was treated as it should be…a dangerous autoimmune disease.

Now…things have changed. Gluten has gone mainstream. Some feel that's a good thing. More publicity means more products, more education, etc, etc. But now, when I try to explain celiac disease, this is what I get: *"Oh…that's that gluten diet thing, right?"* I almost feel the need to defend myself.

What you have done Gwyneth is you have minimized the seriousness of gluten to those who simply cannot have it. Spend a day with me. I'm sure it's not what you go through.

I'm glad you're healthy and happy being gluten-free. I really am. Please just keep it to yourself.

Dean McDermott: A Celiac "Reality" Check

Who is Dean McDermott you say?

If you don't know who is he, then you don't watch reality TV.

And if you don't watch reality TV, then you don't watch "Tori & Dean".

And if you don't watch "Tori & Dean", you are missing some of the best unscripted entertainment the industry has to offer.

Ok…I'm being totally sarcastic. I am not a fan of Reality TV but to each his own.

Alright Gluten Dude…get to the point. What does this have to do with celiac disease?

Well it seems that our friend Dean McDermott has celiac disease. Which in and of itself is not necessarily newsworthy. But whenever a public personality has celiac disease and opens up about it, it can go one of two ways.

Either he/she can become an advocate for the disease and educate people about its implications. Or he/she can mislead the public, making it more difficult for us celiacs to be taken seriously. Since you can tell I'm in a ranting mood, you can guess which route Mr. McDermott decided to take.

Recently, *Allergic Living*, a print magazine dedicated to the celiac community, did an interview with Mr. McDermott about his disease and it was posted on the Celiac Central website.

Here are some lowlights of the interview:

Q: Was it hard to cut gluten out of your diet?
A: I did it slowly. At first, I was eating gluten-free about 50% of the time. So that was easy.

Dude note: Of course it was easy Dean. You didn't make a sacrifice. You didn't do what all celiacs MUST do, which is give up gluten entirely. At this point, the interview should have stopped. It's obvious he doesn't take the disease seriously and a well-known publication should have known he would not be a good advocate. But alas, it proceeded.

Q: Yikes! What does your doctor say about eating gluten occasionally?
A: Since I'm on the low-end of the spectrum, she's not terribly concerned. But I definitely feel better when I'm gluten-free.

Dude note: Kudos to AL for calling him out. But seriously, what the hell?? Celiac disease is not like having the flu. It's an autoimmune disease. This is precisely why celiac disease has become an effing joke in the public eye. And Dean, please do yourself and your intestines a favor and find another doctor. One that won't simply tell you what you want to hear.

Q: How do you avoid eating gluten when you're filming or at press events?
A: People know that I have celiac disease, so they provide gluten-free stuff for me. It can be hard, though. Gluten is used as a thickening agent in sauces and spreads. Unfortunately, I've been gluten-bombed many times.

Dude note: Of course you've been gluten-bombed, Dean. You eat gluten. But hey…it's no big deal. It's not like eating gluten if you have celiac disease can lead to other serious health issues, like cancer. Oh wait…it can lead to cancer? My bad.

To read the rest of the interview, I needed to subscribe to the magazine. Seriously?? After this interview, you expect me to subscribe?

But if I subscribe, I get to read about Dean's plans to open a gluten-free restaurant. I'm assuming only half of the items on the menu will be gluten-free. But you won't know which half. Table for zero please.

Ok, that's enough sarcasm for one post.

I'm just so sick of it all. Sick of the gluten-free celebrities. Sick of the media that covers them. Sick of our plight related to a fad diet.

Addisons. Chrohns. Graves. Lupus. Multiple sclerosis. Rheumatoid arthritis. These are all very serious autoimmune diseases. And they are treated as such, as they should. Just because our disease is food related does not make it any less serious.

But maybe that makes for a boring interview.

My Celiac Plea to Kim Kardashian

The headlines scream. The Twitterverse is abuzz. TMZ is besides themselves. The editors at People Magazine are drooling all over each other.

"KIM KARDASHIAN LOST 6 POUNDS IN SEVEN DAYS BY GIVING UP GLUTEN!"

And celiacs across the world let out a collective groan. Yes, I am paraphrasing a little bit in the headline. She also gave up dairy and sugar. Blogger's prerogative. But I think I speak for most people who have serious gluten issues when I respectfully say this: "Shut the f**k up!"

Do I have a personal bias against her? Perhaps a touch. Her dad helped a murderer get off innocent. She made a sex tape to become famous. She got hitched in a sham marriage for profit. She is the epitome of what is wrong with our celebrity-obsessed culture. But let me take this down a notch and impart a personal plea to Kim.

———

My Dearest Kim,

You are popular. You have a highly-rated TV show. You're on the cover of 97 magazines each week. You have a gazillion followers on Twitter.

Because of this popularity, you can make a difference in people's lives. People, especially susceptible people, will listen to you. And when you say that you can lose weight by going gluten-free, you are sending the wrong message. This is simply, factually untrue.

Giving up gluten has NOTHING to do with weight loss, unless you are replacing those gluten-filled foods with healthy alternatives. But you don't mention that. Your sound bite is simply that you gave up gluten (and dairy and sugar) and it's "HARD!"

But you know what thousands of teenage girls are going to do now? They are going to go gluten-free to lose weight because "that's what Kim did." And then a month from now, I will be in a restaurant and tell the waiter that I cannot have gluten and he will roll his eyes and say "Isn't gluten that thing Kardashian gave up?"

And I will froth at the mouth, steam will come out my ears, my eyes will bulge out of my head, the veins on my forehead will pop and I will say "NO…IT'S POISON TO ME AND ALL PEOPLE WITH CELIAC DISEASE."

But it will fall on deaf ears because you have helped perpetuate the myth that going gluten-free is a surefire way to lose weight. And in two weeks, when you're back to eating gluten again because you didn't realize that gluten is practically in everything and it's too big of a sacrifice, the damage will already have been done. So please Kim…for us celiacs…call your PR company and release another sound bite that goes like this:

"I recently made statements that related giving up gluten to losing weight. I did not realize that gluten can also be very dangerous to those with celiac disease or gluten-sensitivities and I apologize for misleading the public and for making it more difficult for those with celiac disease to be taken seriously. If you want to lose weight, the key is eating healthy and exercising a lot. There are no shortcuts. My apologies to the celiac community."

Thanks for listening Kim.

Gluten Dude

Channing Tatum Goes Gluten-Free. But I Wonder...

It is one of life's complete mysteries why people care what celebrities have to say, like their words have more weight than yours or mine. But it's the world we live in and since they go public with their thoughts, opinions, likes and dislikes, they are fair game. And by the way, I like Mr. Tatum so this is absolutely nothing personal.

Which brings us today to another mindless story about a celebrity going gluten-free to lose weight. In this case, it was Channing Tatum for his role in the film "Magic Mike".

Here is what his publicist said: *"Channing Tatum endured a strict gluten-free diet to prep for the film."*

So...he went strictly gluten-free. Oh I'm sorry, he **endured** going gluten-free (whatever that means). Good for him.

But it does make me wonder a few things...

I wonder if he completely segregated his kitchen to avoid cross-contamination.

I wonder if he asked to speak with the chef every time he went out to eat to make sure his meal was 100% gluten-free.

I wonder if he read food labels on every single item before he purchased them.

I wonder if he called food companies directly when he wasn't sure about an ingredient.

I wonder if he brought his own food with him when going to a friend's house for dinner.

I wonder if he purchased a separate toaster.

I wonder if he made sure every utensil he used went through the dishwasher first.

I wonder if he had to throw away an entire container of butter because there was a crumb in it and he's not sure where it came from.

I wonder if he packed a cooler of food when he was going to be out of the house for the day.

I wonder if he made sure his guests washed their hands before getting ice out of the ice bin.

I wonder if he realized that many people gain weight when they eat gluten-free.

Because you see Channing, for people like us, this is what a strict, gluten-free diet is all about. It sucks. It totally sucks. It's not just the food we give up. We can handle that. It's everything else that goes along with it.

The daily inconveniences. The isolation. The expense.

And when it's all said and done, a lot of us still feel like shit.

But you and your celebrity brethren simply don't understand that. My blog reaches thousands of eyeballs a month. Your ridiculous sound bites reach millions.

And the battle continues...

Finally – A Celebrity Gets Celiac Disease

The title of this article is "Finally…A Celebrity Gets Celiac Disease".

But let me write it a bit more phonetically.

"Finally…A Celebrity **GETS** Celiac Disease."

As in understands; takes it seriously; advocates.

If you've followed this blog for some time (I love you!), you know my relationship with celebrities and gluten/celiac isn't a pretty one. I've railed on Kim Kardashian (a few times). I've wondered about Channing Tatum. I've spewed about Miley Cyrus (and the media). I questioned Lady Gaga. I pleaded with Gwyneth Paltrow. And I unloaded against Dean McDermott.

But finally, we have a celebrity with celiac disease who sees this crappy disease with the same eyes that most of us do.

Her name is Jennifer Esposito.

Confession time: Up until a few months ago, I did not know who she was. I do not watch TV unless it involves Jon Stewart or the New York Giants. But this past summer, I was invited to Schar's first U.S. facility opening and it said Jennifer Esposito, who has celiac disease, would be a special guest.

I was interested in hearing her story. I wanted to make sure she would be a good advocate for us; that she really understood the devil in this disease. When she began to speak, I breathed a huge sigh of relief. She began to tell a story of a hospital visit when the staff didn't even know what celiac was.

She said *"We have a lot of work to do."*

Sadly, after what I think was less than a minute, she was done. And the next two hours were spent listening to a bunch of suits verbally orgasm over each other about how awesome Shar and the new facility is. There was not another word spoken about celiac disease.

And I said *"We have a lot of work to do."*

But Jennifer is doing her part and I couldn't be more pleased. (I know…how often do you see me pleased??)

Jennifer had a recent interview with Huffington Post. Here are some of the highlights:

— *"My symptoms were all over the board. From stomach upset, exhaustion, joint pain, sinus infections, dry skin and hair, panic attacks, depression, back pain — the list could go on."*

— *"It took 20-plus years for a proper diagnosis, not to mention countless [...] doctors and specialists. To this day, I still deal with the side effects of being a celiac and repercussions of improperly being diagnosed over the years."*

Dude note: Dang lazy-ass doctors…that's all it is.

— *"When the doctor called me with the results, she said 'You have the highest case of celiac disease I have ever seen, and I don't know how you are existing.'"*

— *"There is a misconception that if you remove gluten from your diet, you dramatically feel better. This is not true. Yes, many of the stomach issues and other ailment start to subside, but this is an autoimmune disease. Like any other autoimmune disease, it needs your attention every day!"*

Dude note: As a fellow celiac, YES! The mainstream opinion seems to be if we eat gluten-free, we're fine. That's what I thought upon my diagnosis. But as story after story on this blog can attest to, that just ain't the truth.

— *"I am determined to educate and make people aware of the truth about this disease."*

— *"I believe that the medical industry needs to focus on treating the individual person, the whole person, body and mind and not about money and mass studies of a disease."*

— *"For a full-blown celiac patient there is no magic pill for this disease, not even a gluten-free diet. You must constantly be aware of what you are eating and maintain a healthy lifestyle."*

— *"Now we are also faced with a bigger problem. Gluten-free dieting is becoming a fad thanks to high-profile individuals who are removing gluten to achieve weight loss. This makes me want to scream! Going gluten-free may be a trend now, but there is a medical need, a dependency on being careful about not eating gluten and having meals properly prepared to prevent cross-contamination for the millions of people [who] have to deal with celiac disease. I've experienced odd looks at me from wait staff when I say I need my meal to be completely gluten-free with a "yeah right" kind of attitude now. People are becoming cavalier about gluten-free, because they believe it's the new quick fix to getting skinny. Well for the people whose lives depend on it to live, let's just say we are not too happy about this."*

Dude note: Is it possible to love somebody you've never met??

So my fellow celiacs, let us welcome Jennifer into our community with extremely open arms. Let's work together to continue to be the best damn celiac advocates that we can be. Let's join hands in denigrating the gluten-free diet and putting the focus back on the disease itself where it belongs.

And to you Jennifer I say this: I'm sorry you've been afflicted with this disease. It's a journey I wouldn't wish on anyone. But by playing the advocate instead of the victim; by taking it seriously instead of half-ass; by going public instead of staying quiet; you are doing more good than you could ever imagine and hopefully that will give you as much satisfaction than a closet-full of Emmys and Oscars.

Dr. Oz Calls Gluten-Free a Scam

Oh geez. Here we go.

I was never a big fan of Dr. "the sky is falling and I'm making millions off of spreading fear" Oz. He's a smart guy but spends too much time spewing nonsense for ratings. In the past five years on his show, he has shared no less than 16 "miracle weight loss cures". Crap from green coffee extract to raspberry ketone. He offers false hope to millions who are looking for a quick fix.

Hey Dr. Oz…I've got an idea. How about offering the truth that it's a combination of eating right and exercising regularly? Offering the truth? Now that would be a miracle…but wouldn't make for great TV now would it?

So anyway, last night he was on with Seth Myers and for some reason, they just HAD to talk about gluten. What is it with late-night comedians and gluten? Is there nothing else to talk about? Anyway, here is how the conversation went:

Seth: I feel like there are all of these crazes in health and one of these is gluten-free. So gluten-free, is it the real deal or is it BS? What do you think?

Now at this point, I'm thinking Dr. Oz, you know…being a DOCTOR and all, would say it's a real health issue for a lot of people and would go on to talk about celiac disease. I mean this is a real moment to educate. We can finally shut the naysayers up. Jimmy Kimmel, Rachael Ray, Jimmy Fallon and all the other idiots who pile on us can all suck it. This is our moment to shine.

I hit pause on my DVR. I woke my entire family up and told them to come downstairs. I called the neighbors and had them come over. I called all my friends and relatives and put them all on speakerphone so everyone could finally hear from a real doctor about how serious our disease is. I opened all of the windows in my house and turned the volume all the way up.

Then when I had everyone's rapt attention…I hit the play button.

And this is what I got.

Dr. Oz: It's complete BS. It's a scam.

Ok…that's not what I was expecting. And what he said that, the crowd cheered. It's like they were all saying "I KNEW IT!" and they were so deliriously happy.

After he called it a scam, he seemed to try to go into damage control mode a bit but he even botched that. He said "there are a lot of folks who have big time problem with gluten so I don't have a problem with people who don't like eating gluten foods."

We don't LIKE to eat gluten foods? Really?? It's not that we CAN'T eat gluten foods or our body actually attacks itself causing ungodly health issues? Ok, just wanted to make sure.

He finishes nicely, saying that most gluten-free food is junk. Been saying that for years.

And THAT'S what the scam is. It's the food companies promoting gluten-free like it's better for everyone's general health, regardless of how much other crap ingredients they put in their food.

His intent most likely was not to discredit the gluten-free community, but his messaging was atrocious. And naturally…not one mention of celiac disease. Another missed opportunity.

But you know what my real problem with this segment is? Dr. Oz is constantly talking about the evils of gluten on his show and on his site. You want some headlines from the man himself? How about these for starters?

"5 Hidden Signs You Have a Gluten Allergy"

"The New Warning Signs for Gluten Sensitivity"

"Gluten: The Next Epidemic?"

"Is Gluten Your Body's Worst Enemy?"

"Is Gluten Secretly Destroying Your Health?"

"Have You Gone Gluten-Free?"

"Is Going Gluten-Free the Answer You've Been Waiting For?"

See the double-standard here? Dr. Oz can't stop talking about gluten. He's profiting handsomely from it. He's one of the reasons for the damn bandwagon in the first place. And yet he goes on national TV and then calls it complete BS?? You cannot have it both ways, my friend. And the next time a celiac gets sick because a chef thinks the whole gluten-free thing is a scam, he/she will have you to thank.

Well done, Doc.

I'll finish with this wonderful quote from Forbes magazine:

"Dr. Oz simply masquerades marketing as medicine, trumpeting outlandish claims on the backs of poorly conducted science and insignificant data. In the end, it's all for ratings."

Amen to that.

Why the Jimmy Kimmel Video Matters

2017 Gluten Dude: This is regarding a video that Jimmy Kimmel did on his show that made fun of "gluten-free" and went really, really viral.

I promise…this is not going to be a Kimmel-bashing post. Just hang with me.

You would not believe the number of people who contacted me, both publicly and privately, about a video Kimmel showed last night. So I suppose it is my duty to at least broach the subject.

For those who have not seen the video, Jimmy went to the streets and asked people who were gluten-free if they knew what gluten was and then before the person answered, the audience guessed if the person actually knew what gluten was.

Here's something I just picked up on this morning by the way. For the two white people, the audience guessed Yes. For the two minorities, the audience guessed NO. Just an observation…and a bit of a disturbing one at that.

Anyway, the segment was predictable. The four people had no clue. Perhaps they interviewed 100 and only found 4 who didn't know what it was and made it seem like everyone they talked to had no clue. Who knows and who cares.

There are a few reasons the video didn't raise my ire like some of the Jimmy Fallon segments.

First…he did mention that some people have a medical issue with gluten. I seriously just wished he mentioned "Celiac Disease"…just this one time.

Secondly…it makes the idiots who go gluten-free half-ass for all the wrong reasons…well…look like idiots. And I'm all for that.

So even though some in the community were looking to me to call him out, I was going to take a pass. I honestly wasn't offended by the video and my focus this month is on helping people and I didn't want to lose that focus.

But then a few things happened and I realized that maybe the video does matter. And it does affect our community. And by ignoring it, I'm not doing my job. (Well…a job actually pays but you know what I mean.)

So what happened? Let me explain:

1) We became a running joke on Twitter all day yesterday. People were sharing the video link left and right with comments like *"See? Gluten-free people don't even know what gluten is!"* and *"I knew gluten-free was complete BS."* and on and on. And any time the focus switches from "gluten-free is a medical necessity" to "gluten-free isn't real", it hurts our cause. We get taken less seriously.

2) I received the following email a few weeks ago from someone whose life is in absolute shambles because of what is most likely undiagnosed celiac and it spoke of the Hollywood connection.

> ''
>
> When I was a boy of only six tender years, I was baptized into the fold of chronic disease sufferers. I had asthma. Asthma is an invisible condition. Unless one has an attack within the near proximity of another, the second person might never know of its existence. And what does that lead to? Doubt. Disbelief.
>
> From a young age I was frequently told that my illness was all in my head. Adults told me this. My gym teacher told me this. I was teased and accused of laziness and attention-seeking behavior.

What made all of this worse, of course, was that Hollywood would help propagate this myth. In how many movies, especially during those horrible 1980s, was the nerd, the dork, or the loser shown to use an inhaler?

Celiac is the same, of course. It has been granted the same protection in Hollywood and on television. It's sufferers have been deemed fodder for insult, doubt and accusations. It's despicable, and it leads to all sorts of socially acceptable behavior that is not tolerated for other diseases.

After years of varying symptoms, I visited my doctor. He doubted my symptoms and accused me of faking illness to get out of work. He refused to sign a release that would have essentially forgiven my level of absenteeism. He refused further treatment and sent me back to work.

The following day, I again became violently sick and had to ask to go home. I was fired on my way out.

Last year, two of my siblings were both diagnosed with Celiac Disease after suffering similar ailments. Their conditions were verified with the genetic tests and intestinal biopsies. Additionally, cancers of the bowel and digestive system run in one side of the family, which further lends credence to the belief.

I assume I have the disease, and have experienced some level of recovery since giving up gluten and its substitutes for the last five months. I mention all of this because all of this could have been prevented if my doctor would have simply done his job, or failing that, referred me to a doctor who would have done his or her job. It is ironic to me that the man who ruined my life accused me of not wanting to do my job when he clearly had no inclination to do his own.

"

Right or wrong, Hollywood has power. What they say matters in the country. So here's my question. Would doctors be more apt to test for celiac and take it seriously if gluten-free wasn't such a big joke? If people like Kimmel and Fallon and Meyers would just lay off the jokes, or at least mention celiac disease, couldn't they be part of the solution instead of part of the problem?

You know who never makes fun of the gluten-free fad? Jon Stewart. Why? One…because he's not a lazy comedian. And two…because his wife has celiac disease. You think if Kimmel's wife had celiac, he'd change his tune a little? Yeah…me too.

It's so easy to make fun of something when it doesn't affect you directly. Pathetic but true.

3) As I'm writing this post, I received the following message on Facebook. It is from a fellow celiac in Australia and it seems like the bullying trend is making its way overseas.

> ❝
>
> Just wondering if you have seen the Jimmy Kimmel show? Taking a pot shot at gluten free people who don't know what it is and how annoying coeliacs are. What is it with you guys in America? It kind of seems like the shows there like to bully people. And the trend is catching on here too. We have a stupid show called The Project and they had a crack at coeliacs the other day. Dude, I didn't know how bad you had it over there and I feel for you all. Keep fighting the good fight. Xxxxx
>
> ❞

Is there a connection between the gluten-free jokes and the lack of celiac awareness? Am I stretching things a bit? I really don't know. You tell me.

Look, we need laughter in this world. We need it desperately. And believe it or not, I'm a big fan of Kimmel, Fallon and Meyers.

All I'm asking is that they lay off the gluten-free jokes a bit. Let the nation move onto to something else. So the celiac community can be taken seriously again. So our words are listened to when we are in a restaurant. So our doctors put celiac at the top of their list when diagnosing someone with a variety of seemingly unrelated symptoms.

Then, when the dust settles, run that video again and I'll laugh my ass off. What a bunch of boneheads.

A Conversation with Jennifer Esposito: Actress and Fellow Celiac Advocate

2017 Gluten Dude: If you have not read Jennifer's book (*My Journey with Celiac Disease*), I strongly suggest it. Her story is one to be read and she's got some great advice that you won't hear in many other places and some excellent recipes to boot.

On TV, Jennifer Esposito has acted in popular TV shows such as Spin City, Law and Order, Rescue Me, Samantha Who and Blue Bloods. On film, she has worked on great films such as Summer of Sam, Crash and Wes Craven's Dracula:2000.

But in real life, Jennifer has another role: celiac advocate. In the following interview, she shares her thoughts on her career, her diagnosis and her passion about celiac disease.

Enjoy!

GD: I'll start off with a non-celiac question. Back in my 20's, I was an actor. Studied with some great teachers; lived in both NYC and Los Angeles; got some spots on soap operas and independent films. But by and large, I was a spectacular failure. I tried telling myself the acting gods just weren't with me. But I think mostly I was just a crappy actor. What do you attain your success to?

JE: There were two things I loved as a child: eating and entertaining. When I wasn't making a mess in the kitchen trying to create some delicious goodies, I was that annoying child putting on plays, dancing, even walking and flipping myself off the couch into company that was sitting there. Basically anyone who stood still for more than 2 minutes would have to endure some kind of performance by me.

251

As I got older acting became my love. When I started working professionally I was told everything from your too ethnic, your not ethnic enough, you sound like from your from NY, your teeth aren't straight and was even told my a few agents "I don't get it" IT meaning ME. The reason for my success as you asked, sheer perseverance. I'm not good with people telling me who and what I am, as well as telling me how and what I can do with my life.

GD: And a follow up question. Pursuing an acting career can be a brutal experience. Given all of your health woes, how the heck did you maintain your energy and your sanity while following your dream?

JE: To say the business is brutal is an absolute understatement. Don't get me wrong, I did not make it to this point unscathed. The pressure and constant battle to prove myself as an actress in the entertainment business took a major toll on me; leading me to many many years of struggle personally, emotionally, spiritually and yes physical.

Never realizing that contributing to this struggle was emanating from a hidden disease. My undiagnosed Celiac took many shapes and forms regarding my health mentally and physically. Falling asleep on any break I ever had while filming was normal for me. Makeup artists dealing with my yellow skin (due to constant elevated liver enzymes from the disease) leading me to always bring a specially formulated color foundation that matched my skin. Depression and anxiety that shaped my every day.

Also being told I had an attitude from producers at times because I sometimes would get really quiet from exhaustion, stomach issue and anxiety attacks. People would think that after 20+ years in the business, 15 movies, countless TV shows and even awards would somehow make this business easier.

WRONG!

The discrimination from the business that I am dealing with at this present moment due to this disease is so very sad and completely infuriating. Something I wish I could explain more right now but can't, but be certain that I will in the future.

So hopefully my long winded answer was sufficient but to tie it up, I have absolutely no idea how I have stayed in the business that I'm in so long. I love acting but can't say I love the business.

GD: You tell a very powerful story on your website about how, after an examination where you were hoping to get some answers to all of your health issues, the doctor simply said *"Jennifer, do you want to kill yourself?"* The subtle suggestion by your doctor was that your symptoms were not real…that you were suffering from depression. You tell another story of someone who was on chemotherapy for Crohns disease for TWO YEARS. It turns out, he didn't even have Crohns. He had celiac disease. I have heard horror story after horror story on my blog of people's experiences with their doctors. In your opinion, why is this and what can we do about it?

JF.: Oh goodness, you really want to know what I think regarding why we don't get better attention with this disease???? MONEY. Sorry folks that's what I believe. This disease has NO PILL ANYONE CAN SELL US! This disease is the only disease that can be managed by food alone! That means big financial loss for pharmaceutical companies. Think about the money most of us have spent on these "false diagnoses". I know for me the number is probably close to $500k, between tests, antibiotics, doctor after doctor and then psychotherapists all leading to nothing.

In saying that, are we going to remedy this problem? Probably not. That's why EDUCATION is KEY! If we as the consumer stop buying the processed crap (sorry) that they are selling us, then maybe we will get a change. Maybe.

GD: Most people feel relief when they get diagnosed with celiac disease. Personally, I was pretty angry/resentful. What was your very

first reaction upon learning of your celiac diagnosis? Did you go through any "stages" to get to acceptance?

JE: I personally was overjoyed to hear I had a disease. Reason being because I was told it was in my head and I was crazy for years! I ALWAYS knew that something was wrong. Also at the time of diagnosis I was so severely ill I just wanted some kind of an answer.

I will say until this very day I go through very sad and broken days about this disease. I deal with many other issues due to this disease going undiagnosed for so long and there are days it gets to me. The constant monitoring of EVERYTHING that comes into my surroundings is quite exhausting to say the least.

I do have acceptance of this disease though. It is what it is but as I said earlier I will not let it tell me what and who I am, especially what I can eat. That's why I started baking and cooking like a madman. The thought of NEVER having bread again was something I just couldn't digest, excuse the pun. I will not live in constant deprival of things I love. Everything from bagels, to cupcakes, to pancakes is still all within my reach, just healthier now. Being able to make these things not only quenched my appetite but gave me a sense of control over this consuming disease.

For anyone who has this disease I recommend getting in your kitchen today and taking your life back!

GD: I assume you spend a lot of your time on the road and away from your gluten-free comfort zone. How do you ensure you are safe to eat when you are on movie/TV sets/events for long stretches of time?

JE: I bring a lunchbox wherever I go. When traveling, I always rent somewhere with a kitchen so I don't have to rely on eating out. It's not easy but doable. It's all about planning. When I work long weeks or days, I cook big meals and freeze them and make a muffin of the week to take and snack all the time.

GD: What do you miss the most from your non-celiac days?

JE: Spontaneity. Casually going through your day and stopping for a bite at a new restaurant is something I truly miss. I also LOVE food and loved going to experience what the chef created rather than getting the salad and the plainest of dishes on the menu.

GD: I'm a big believer that "we are what we eat" and that food plays a HUGE part in our overall health. And yet, by and large, we are an incredibly unhealthy society. What can we do to get people to eat healthier without coming across as preachy or controlling?

JE. I think everyone has their own road to go down. All we can do is give people a CHOICE as far as info towards eating well I too completely agree that we are what we eat; unfortunately people don't care enough about themselves sometimes to believe they are worth more. It's also a commitment to really watch what you eat. Everyone is so busy these days they don't believe they have time to eat right. Not so; you are WORTH taking the time to eat well. Believing that is the first step though.

GD: You are out to dinner with Kim Kardashian, Gwyneth Paltrow, Dr. Oz and Dean McDermott. For the main course, your guests all give the waitress a hard time about how the meal must be 100% gluten-free. But then come dessert time, they each order a piece of gluten-filled cake. What, if anything, do you say to them?

JE: Sorry I would have left before appetizers.

Dude Note: LOVE that answer. No wonder we get along so well.

I Just Finished Your Book. Now What?

First...thanks for taking the journey with me. Quite the ride, wasn't it? And I'm sure it will continue to be just as wild on the back nine. The question is...what do you do now?

That's simple.

Eat Right: Take care of your body and your body will take care of you.

Eat Smart: Don't go to a restaurant just because they advertise gluten-free. Be your own best advocate. And if in doubt, do without.

Educate: Make sure the people around you truly know what celiac disease is and how it can affect every fiber of our being.

Connect: Connect with others in the celiac community. It's a pretty cool bunch and you won't feel all alone in this journey.

Advocate: Start a blog. Join a Facebook group. Get active on Twitter. Sadly, the world and even much of the medical community is still pretty ignorant about our autoimmune disease. Let's un-ignorant them. Wait...that's not right. Let's de-ignorantize them. Nope...still doesn't sound right. You get the point.

Laugh: This is the best medicine of all. Don't let people laugh AT you because of celiac disease. But learn to laugh at yourself as much as humanly possible.

And THAT'S all I got (for now). What a long strange trip it's been.

This is Dedicated to the Ones I Love

Special shout outs to some special people who have been a part of my journey.

My parents. One of you most likely passed the celiac gene down to me (but I won't hold you responsible). Thanks for raising me the right way. I just wish you were still around to read this book. I would've even offered you a 50% discount.

My extended family and friends. You make me feel welcome in your homes even though it can be a pain in the ass. You go out of your way to keep me safe. You make me feel like I'm just a normal guy…and not a celiac. For that, I am forever grateful.

The celiac community. You opened your arms to me and allowed me to be a "voice" within the community. I thank you for that. Except for the one who called me Gluten Douche. That was hurtful (but serious kudos for originality.)

Alysa Bajenaru. You are a helpful ear when I'm struggling. Knowing I can send you a text that says "celiac sucks" once in a while and the fact that you "get it" has been a blessing. Maybe one day, we'll actually meet! *(Dude note: If you don't have a fellow celiac that you can lean on like this…find one.)*

Jennifer Esposito. You are my celiac sister and fellow passionate advocate who puts the celiac community first every single time. Oh yeah…and an actress and a best-selling author. And don't even get me started on your baked goods & recipes. Oh my!!! Jen…seriously so glad you are in mine and Mrs. Dude's life.

The Dudettes. You learned on day one (and you were YOUNG) what was dangerous to me and what was safe. You didn't complain. You didn't blink. Dang impressive. And you haven't wavered in your support and love. Ever. Love you both to the moon and back.

Mrs. Dude. What can I say that I haven't said a hundred times in my blog? You are my rock. You are my best friend. You are my partner in this crazy journey called life. Words are not enough to show my gratitude. Love you more than you will ever know. Sushi tonight??